MW00462519

Korean Medicine

A Holistic Way to Health and Healing

KOREA ESSENTIALS No. 14

Korean Medicine: A Holistic Way to Health and Healing

Published in 2013 by Seoul Selection
B1 Korean Publishers Association Bldg., 105-2 Sagan-dong, Jongno-gu,
Seoul 110-190, Korea
Phone: (82-2) 734-9567
Fax: (82-2) 734-9562
Email: publisher@seoulselection.com
Website: www.seoulselection.com

ISBN: 978-89-97639-39-7 04080
ISBN: 978-89-91913-70-7 (set)
Printed in the Republic of Korea

Korean Medicine

A Holistic Way to Health and Healing

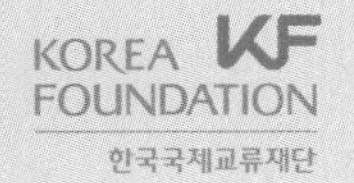

Seoul Selection

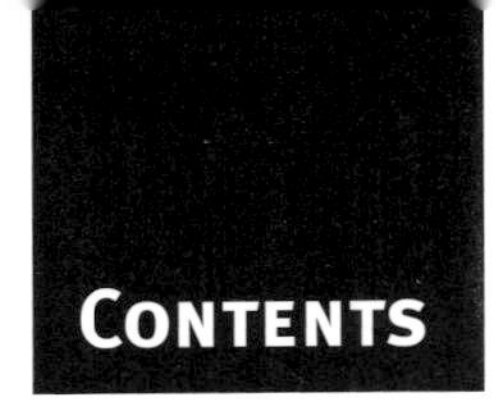
CONTENTS

Delving Deeper

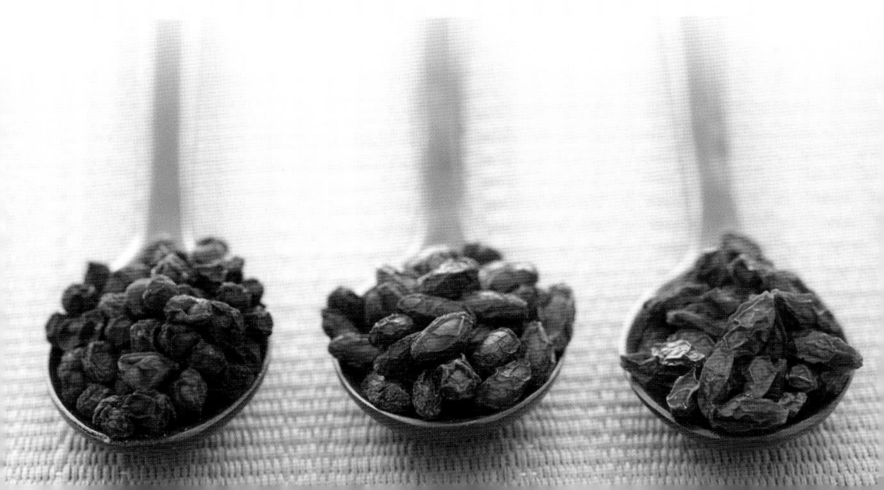

INTRODUCTION

Korean traditional medicine* has long been an important part of Korean culture. Many years before Western medicine arrived in the country, it was used to cure and prevent diseases. Korean traditional medicine went through a period of decline in attention and importance after the arrival of Western medicine, but that has been changing in recent years. More people around the world are growingly aware of the limits of the Western approach and turning to alternative forms of medicine. The U.S. alone has 50 colleges of Oriental medicine, with more to be found in European countries. Interest in acupuncture and herbal treatments is soaring, and as the effectiveness of Korean traditional medicine gets more well known, the numbers of foreigners flocking to clinics has steadily risen.

This book explores Korean traditional medicine in six chapters, examining everything from its origins to present-day forms and potential. In addition to its differences from Western medicine, the basic principles used to understand the patient and diseases will be looked at. Methods of diagnosis and treatment will also be explored. Many know of acupuncture, moxibustion, and herbal remedies, but there are also many other methods; cupping, chuna, aromatherapy, and taping, to name just a few. The book also examines how Korean traditional medicine can be applied to specific conditions and situations, from the common cold to menopausal symptoms, headaches, depression and anger

* Korean medicine is the official English-language name for *haneuihak* as designated by the Association of Korean Medicine and the Korean Medicine Hospitals' Association. This book uses the term "Korean traditional medicine" to avoid confusion with Western medicine as practiced in Korea.

management, fatigue, pregnancy and childbirth, postpartum treatment, and even hair loss. Finally, the last section will describe how Korean traditional medicine is moving beyond Korea's borders to reach people all around the world. Interspersed with all of this are brief sidebars on topics such as *Donguibogam,* a text known as the bible of Korean traditional medicine; *sasang* (four physical constitutions) medicine, an unique concept that sets the Korean approach apart from other forms of Oriental medicine; the use of acupuncture in the ear to help people quit smoking; steam bidet therapy used to apply herbal treatment externally; Korea's storied herbal markets; and the most frequently used herbs.

The intent of this book is to help Korean traditional medicine become more accessible to foreign readers and help people around the world live a more healthy, disease-free life thanks to Korea's outstanding medical know-how.

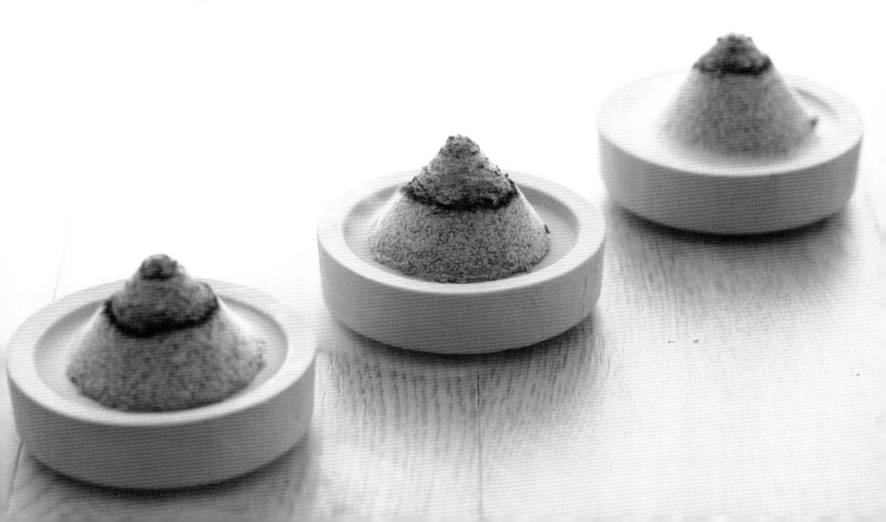

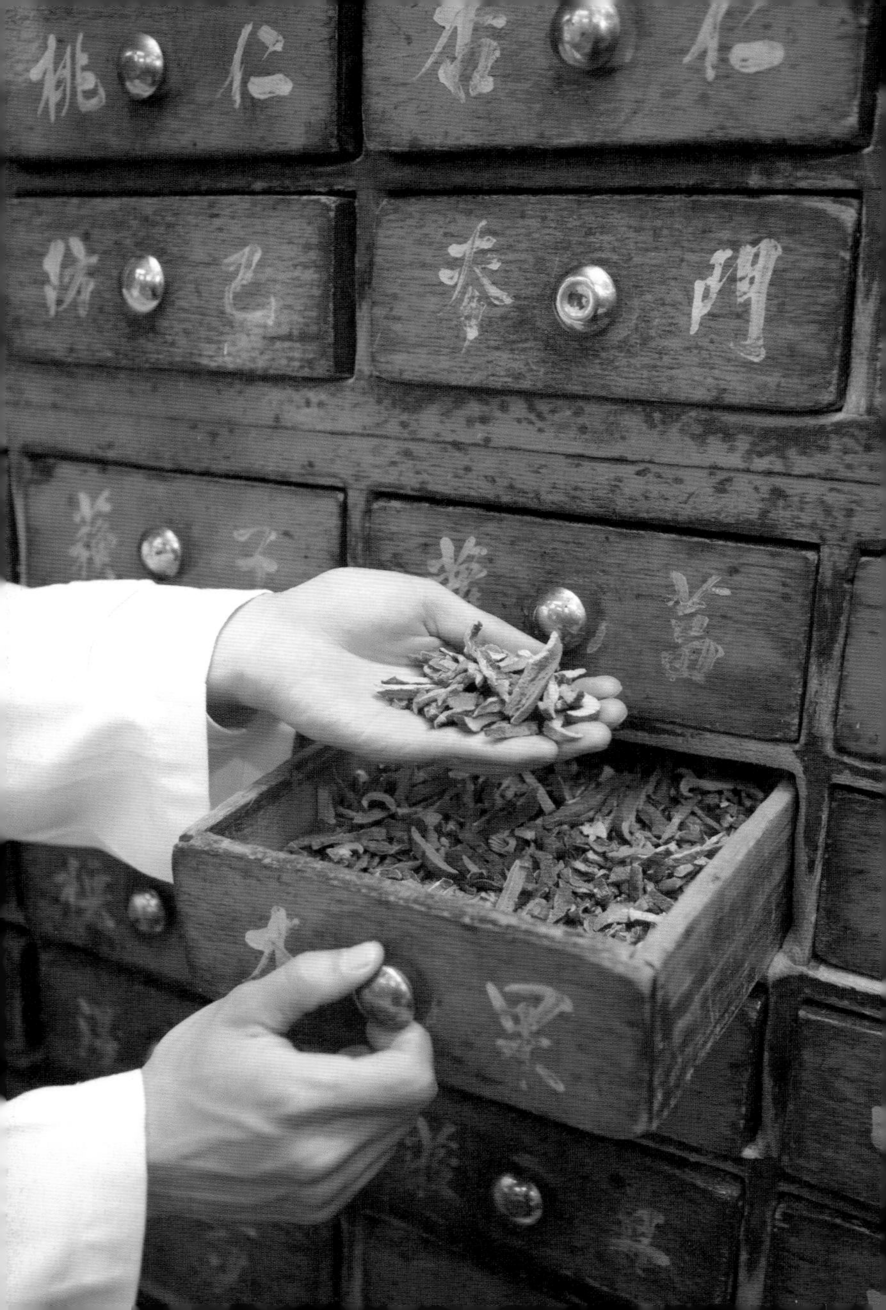
桃仁
防己

"The physician should not treat the disease
but the patient who is suffering from it."

– Maimonides

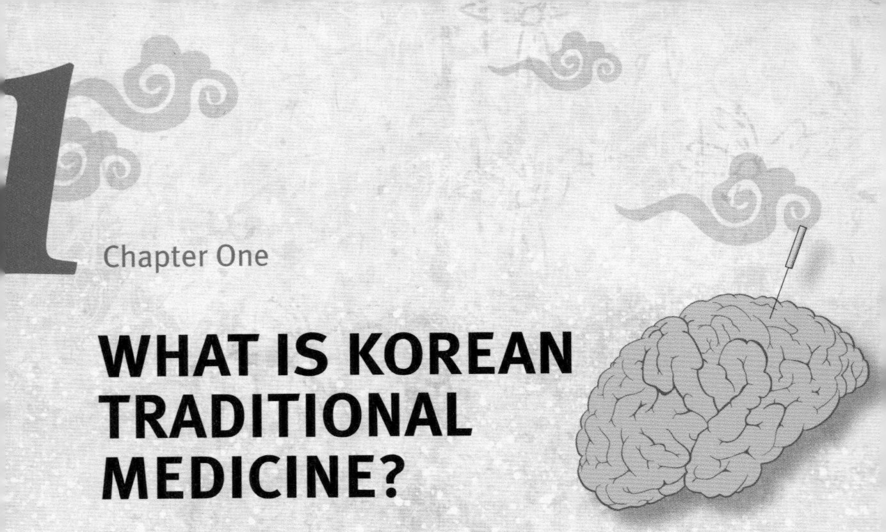

Chapter One

WHAT IS KOREAN TRADITIONAL MEDICINE?

ORIGINS AND HISTORY

Korean traditional medicine has developed with the Korean people, and is a product of their collective wisdom. Although ancient Koreans are known to have learned much from neighboring countries such as China, they developed their own medicine better suited to their lifestyle and physical constitution rather than simply following the Chinese model.

Ancient Times

From the time the first people arrived on the Korean Peninsula, Koreans have continuously developed and refined their medical knowledge. Early on, this was related mainly to remedial treatment such as easing pain or tending to injury, along with knowing what foods were good for health. In particular, due to its powerful influence, nature became an object of worship and ritual practices. This animistic belief later evolved into shamanism, which reinforced the notion that all things have a spirit. Related to this, a physical ailment was thought to be caused by the influence of evil spirits, for which a shaman was needed to provide a remedy.

Evidence of ancient Korean medicine can be found in the Dangun myth, in which mugwort and garlic were prescribed. The Dangun creation myth, which is said to recount the origin of the Korean people, was recorded in several historical journals, including "Memorabilia of the Three Kingdoms (*Samgukyusa*)," which was written during the Goryeo Dynasty period (918–1392). This account of the birth of the original Korean nation, Old Joseon (2333–108 B.C.), tells of a bear and tiger who, after appealing to the gods to allow them to take on human form, were told to eat mugwort and garlic.

Medicine chest with names indicating which medicine goes in each drawer

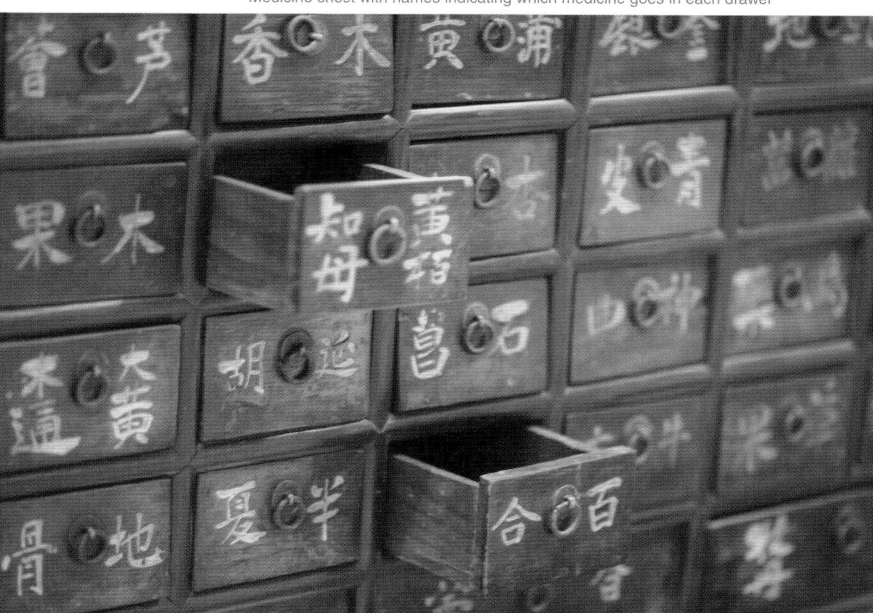

This provides insight into how ancient Koreans recognized the efficacy of herbal medicine. Even the foremost Chinese medical journal, *Shen Nong Ben Cao Jing* (Shen Nong Materia Medica), contained no reference to mugwort or garlic. Compiled in the Later Han Dynasty (25–220) and the Three Kingdoms period (220–280) of China, this journal describes the uses for 365 medicines. The lack of any reference to mugwort or garlic seems to verify the independent development of Korean traditional medicine.

In Korea's Three Kingdoms period (57 B.C.– A.D. 668), significant exchanges were conducted with other countries, to the point that such foreign influences eventually permeated Korean culture and medicine. In particular, medical knowledge from China and India supplemented the foundation of traditional medicine in Korea that had been handed down from the Old Joseon period, which spurred further development.

This trend continued into the Unified Silla period (676–935), with Korean medicine being blended with those of China and India and then localized. In the Goryeo period (918–1392), a variety of medicinal ingredients were introduced to Korea by China's Song Dynasty (960–1279) as well as Arab merchants, and this contributed to the expansion of Korea's medical knowledge.

Origins of the Korean Approach

Korea began to establish a truly unique form of traditional medicine in the Goryeo Dynasty period due primarily to the lack of development of Chinese medicine after the founding of the Yuan Dynasty (1271–1368) and subsequent decline in the value of Sino-Korean medical exchanges. So a Korean form of medicine tailored to Korea's conditions began to thrive, and this included the publication of medical journals, such as *Jejungiphyobang* (An Introductory Guide to Medicine for the General Public), *Eouichwal yobang* (The Essential Guide to Mastering Medicine), and

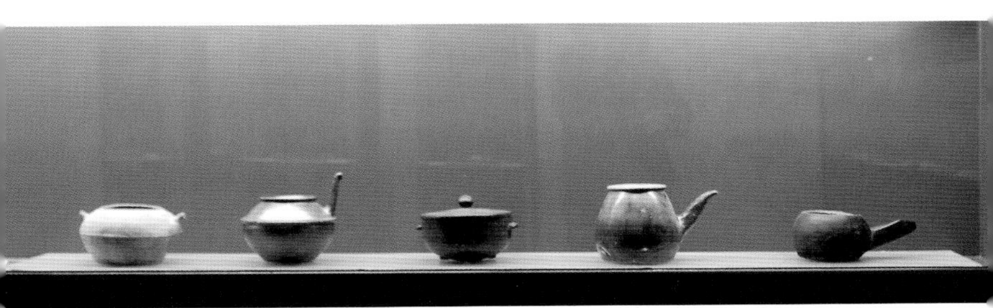

Display of old medicine brewing pot at the Choonwondang Museum of Korean Medicine that were used to brew or heat herbal concoctions

Hyangyakgugeupbang (Guide to Korean Medicine and First Aid). These publications included medical knowledge from China's Song and Yuan dynasties and elsewhere, but also documented extensive research findings of medicinal ingredients indigenous to Korea. They also showed the significant advancement of Korean traditional medicine from the Old Joseon period.

The uniqueness of Korean traditional medicine, which had emerged in the late Goryeo period, continued through the Joseon period (1392–1910). For example, the first training system for nurses was instituted under Joseon Dynasty King Taejong (r. 1400–1418), while under King Sejong's reign (r. 1418–1450) measures were adopted to promote the development of a variety of Korean medicinal ingredients. These efforts were systematized and published in *Hyangyakjipseongbang* (A Cumulative Guide to Korean Medicine).

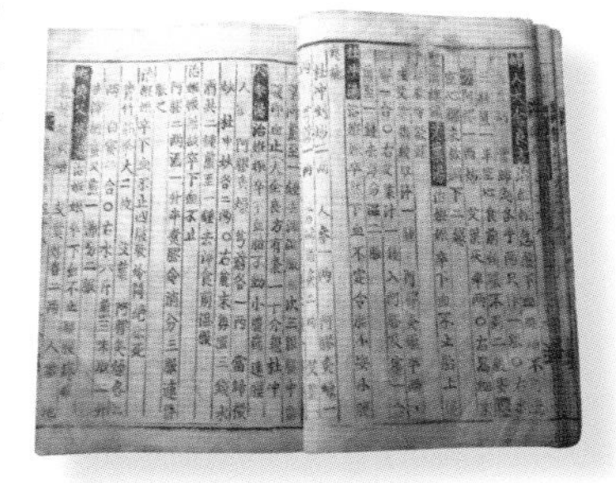

Hyangyakjipseongbang

In addition, exchange between Korea and China continued, which had an effect on the development of medical research in Korea. The results

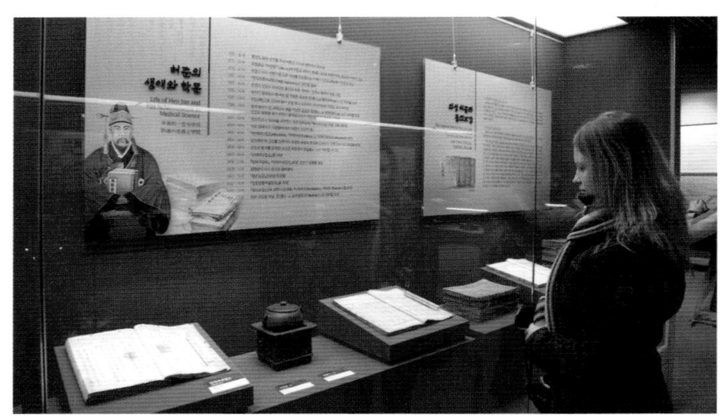

A visitor looks at exhibits on Korean medicine pioneer Heo Jun and The *Donguibogam* at Sancheong Museum of Herbal Medicine.

of this research were published in *Uibangyuchwi* (Classification of the Medical Arts). Thereafter, several medical journals were introduced from Ming Dynasty China (1368–1644) while specialized medical texts including detailed accounts of clinical research were also written in Korea.

In the mid-Joseon period, the scholar Heo Jun (1539–1615) compiled *Donguibogam* (Principles and Practices of Korean Medicine), which is considered one of the most outstanding achievements in Oriental medicine. Comprising a summary of Oriental medicine based on Korean traditional medicine and a medical text that systematized concepts handed down from generation to generation, the book was widely distributed throughout Korea, China, and Japan, and is used as a reference even today.

In the late Joseon period of the 19th century, greater emphasis was placed on practicality, leading to the emergence of positivistic schools of thought and, in turn, the categorization and specialization of knowledge. As such, treatment methods that were practical and convenient in everyday life were promoted to improve the welfare of the common people.

Around this time, Yi Jema developed a unique system of *sasang* medicine ("medicine of the four physical constitutions"), which best exemplifies the indigenous nature of Korean traditional medicine. In this innovative system, people were categorized into four types of physical constitutions. At that time, medical treatment was based on the principles of *yin* and *yang* and the five elements, such that a "*yin*" person would be prescribed a treatment of warmth, and a "*yang*" person treated with cold. Yi opened a new horizon in Korean medicine by first determining a person's constitution type, then diagnosing the problem and prescribing the most appropriate treatment.

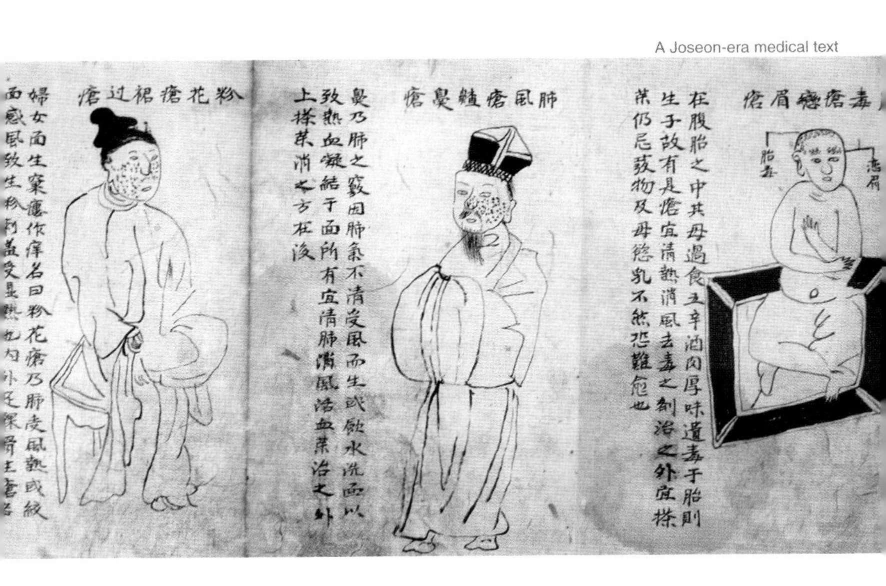

A Joseon-era medical text

Donguibogam: The World's First Medical Text for Laypeople

Donguibogam was the result of a collaborative effort launched in 1596. Korea had just repelled a Japanese invasion in the so-called Imjin War, and an array of luminaries including Heo Jun, Jeong Jak, Yang Ye-su, Kim Eung-tak, Lee Myeong-won, and Jeong Ye-nam, were appointed to write a text on the development of disease treatment and medical techniques. But the peace did not last long. The following year, Japan made another invasion attempt in what is called the Jeongyu War. The writing project was put on hold, and Heo was later ordered to finish the book by himself. He set up an editorial board within the royal medical center, and in August 1610 (the second year of the reign of King Gwanghae), the 25-book set was complete 14 years after the project was started.

Donguibogam differs from other medical books in organization. Whereas previous books had been classified by disease, Heo's methods were more akin to those of modern clinical medicine. His book was divided into five sections: the first on internal medicine (*naegyeongpyeon*); the second on external medicine, ophthalmology, otorhinolaryngology, dermatology, and urology (*oehyeongpyeon*); the third on pathology, diagnosis, allopathy, emergency treatment, epidemiology, obstetrics, and pediatrics (*japbyeongpyeon*); the fourth on clinical pharmacology (*tangaekpyeon*); and the fifth on meridian points and acupuncture (*chimgupyeon*).

This structure shows the way Korean medicine emphasizes prevention over treatment; the shape of the body, pathological conditions, and principles of disease are explained first, and only afterwards are the procedures for herbal treatment and acupuncture described. Similarly, the most common conditions are generally dealt

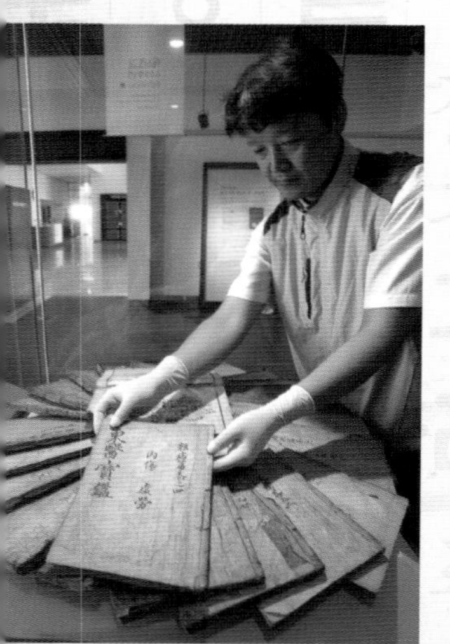

The mammoth *Donguibogam* comprises 25 volumes.

with first, and descriptions of symptoms are organized to make it easy to find the causes, make a diagnosis, and offer the appropriate remedy. The prescriptions are given in detail and exhaustively sourced, with occasional references to folk remedies and "secret methods" from the author's own experiences to help promote the effectiveness of the treatments.

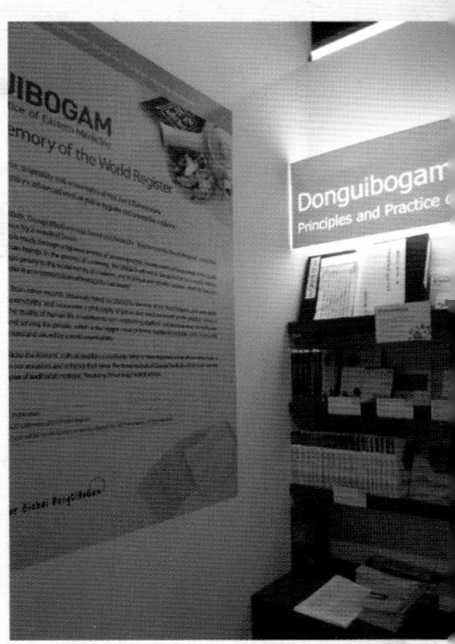

Exhibit on the *Donguibogam* for the Korea Pavilion at the 2009 Frankfurt Book Fair

Donguibogam is more than just a clinical text. It incorporates all of the basic theories of Chinese medicine along with methods and herbs unique to Korea. This comprehensive compendium of Korean medical knowledge is a veritable encyclopedia of East Asian medicine and the world's first medical text for the general public. The herbs described by the authors were not expensive Chinese imports, but things that Korean readers could find relatively easily, and their names are given both in the specialized terminology of clinics and the vernacular terms used by the public. The book's excellence was recognized in 2009 when it became the first medical text to earn designation on UNESCO's Memory of the World Register.

Author Heo Jun (1539–1615) was a Joseon-era medical officer not only highly skilled in treatment but also deeply devoted to medical study and widely trusted by the kings he served, Seonjo and Gwanghae. Heo wrote a number of other medical texts, including two on infectious diseases, *Sinchanbyeogonbang* and *Byeogyeoksinbang*. He also promoted their use by a wider public by translating them from Chinese into regular Korean script, a contribution that helped tremendously in the academic and scientific development of Korean medicine. An advocate of empirical study, Heo was a gifted observer who brought a profound understanding of the classics to the field of clinical medicine, helping to create a framework that was both systematic and practical. In addition to influencing future generations of physicians, he laid the groundwork for medicine to reach the public. His contribution was truly a turning point in the history of Korean medicine.

The Wave of the Future

Amid the introduction of Western medicine and Japanese colonial rule (1910–1945), Korean traditional medicine fell on hard times. Imperial Japan's efforts to eradicate Korean culture, as well as Korea's traditional medicine, led to a 40-year suspension of academic research and development of traditional medicine in Korea.

Shortly after this period of suppression ended with Korea's liberation from Japanese rule, the National Medical Treatment Law was enacted in 1951, which established a system for practitioners of traditional medicine supported by the government and the public. And by the 1970s, the value of Korean traditional medicine such as acupuncture was widely recognized by medical clinics, along with a diverse range of academic research being undertaken in this field.

The theme of the 2013 Korean Medicine-Bio Fair in Jecheon was "Making Korean Medicine Commercial, Scientific, and Global."

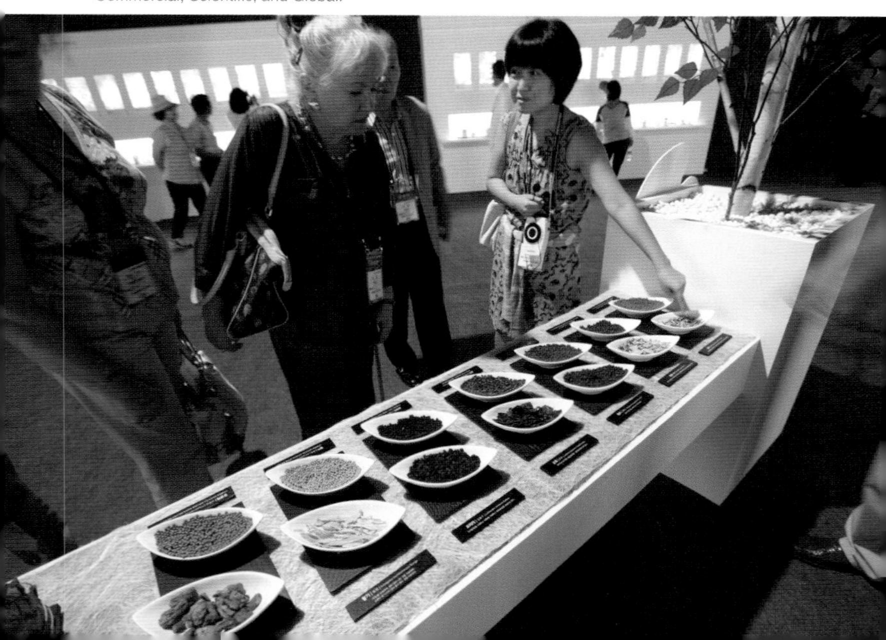

In response to growing global interest in traditional medicine, the World Health Organization has been sponsoring studies of traditional medicine in other countries, including efforts to designate international standards for acupuncture. In 1987, Korea hosted an international conference for the purpose of promoting standardized terminology for traditional medicine.

With the foundation of the Korea Institute of Oriental Medicine in 1994, the Korean government adopted an institutional framework for the promotion of Korean traditional medicine and support for related research activities. Today, 11 specialized colleges are leading the way in actively advancing the applications and technology of Korean traditional medicine.

Differences from Western Medicine

Korean and Western medicine both seek to treat ailments. Their goal is the same: keep people healthy. But they differ greatly in how they view and treat symptoms and sicknesses.

In Korean traditional medicine, the body is seen as part of nature and the cosmos, but one that is its own microcosm that constantly interacts with nature. So the approach to understanding the body is mainly philosophical and steeped in metaphysics. This contrasts with Western medicine's view of the body as something separate and independent from nature, where the primary emphasis is analyzing and understanding it in terms of its anatomical organization.

Given these differences in views, it should come as no surprise that they differ in what is considered "disease." Korean traditional medicine believes that disease is present whenever a person feels not healthy—in other words, when symptoms are present—regardless of any organic changes that might or might not have occurred. For example, a patient could feel tired, not hungry, or enervated though an examination finds no problems. Seemingly trivial complaints like a constricted feeling in the chest and unexplained feeling of anxiety are all understood to be signs of disease.

The diagnoses of Western medicine, in contrast, emphasize organic changes under the idea that when these changes are corrected or removed, the patient will get healthier. If a patient's inflammation, paralysis, sensory disturbances (hallucinations or pain), or tumor goes away, then he or she is seen as cured, whatever the complaint. Recently, Western medicine has been focusing more on functional disorders like indigestion and chronic fatigue syndrome that arise despite no signs of structural problems. But in most cases, a complaint is not viewed as subject to treatment unless it meets the quantifiable diagnostic standards of a given ailment.

This fundamental difference has shaped the development of the two approaches. Korean traditional medicine focuses more on the patient's perceived health, while Western medicine tries to eliminate things that cause disease.

Those causes are another area in which the two approaches differ. Practitioners of Korean traditional medicine say the ultimate cause of disease is not so much the intrusion of external elements, but malfunctions in inherent bodily function. Since diseases are considered to result from the patient's own enfeeblement or the weakening of his or her vital energy, the emphasis is on boosting the body's ability to defend against them. Illnesses may be attributed to emotional states like joy or sorrow, or other internal causes such as overwork and fluctuations in internal organ functions. Even diseases that appear to have external causes are ultimately seen as the products of internal factors. If one's ability to fend off sickness is strong enough, one will not get sick even if pathogens do enter the body. Thus, treatment is focused mainly on bolstering the body's own vital energy.

Western medicine, on the other hand, looks mainly at anatomical causes. It looks for external pathogens like viruses and bacteria that have entered the body and impaired tissues. Treatment, as a rule, is focused on ridding the body of these pathogens.

Because Korean traditional medicine emphasizes internal causes, the patient rather than the physician is seen as being responsible for treatment. The physician's job is to help the patient strengthen his or her own immune functions; ultimately, the patient can achieve good health through proper diet, sleep habits, and daily routine. In this, Korean traditional medicine differs from the Western approach, where the active role belongs to a skilled physician who treats a comparatively passive patient.

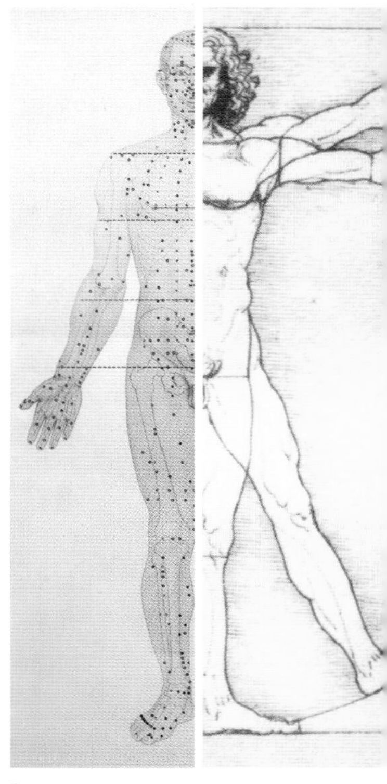

East and West have traditionally held different views on the human body and health. The Western schema shows attention to anatomical detail with each muscle indicated, while the one for Oriental medicine lists meridians and acupuncture points.

Despite these differences, more emphasis on recent years has been placed on the commonalities and places where the two approaches intersect. Korean traditional medicine's emphasis on fighting "bad energy" with vital energy, for example, overlaps in many ways with Western medicine's explanation of disease in terms of immune functions and responses. Similarly, the constitutional medicine approach, which considers individual characteristics and physical makeup, can be tied to contemporary studies on the genome.

Korean, Chinese and Japanese Traditions in Medicine

The Chinese medical tradition dates back thousands of years, and its influence on Korea, Japan, and other countries all over Asia has been profound. Korean traditional medicine is fundamentally rooted in this approach, but has also developed independently in the centuries since the Joseon Dynasty. The first real development of a distinctive Korean medicine can be traced to the early Joseon period, when ancient indigenous methods of treatment were compiled into a text called *Hyangyakjipseongbang*. But the later publication of *Uibangyuchwi*, East Asia's first medical encyclopedia, allowed the framework of Korean traditional medicine to truly take shape. This book was followed by Heo Jun's *Donguibogam* and Yi Je-ma's *Donguisusebowon*, which articulated the basic principles of the constitutional medicine approach known as *sasang* ("four constitutional forms"). By this point, Korean traditional medicine was developing its own tradition distinct from China's and focused on the human body's constitutional characteristics and connection with nature, a "human-centered" approach to medicine, one might say. Its research approach was grounded in the Neo-Confucian tradition and a philosophy of "serving the multitude," and the emphasis was on internal causes and experience-based approaches.

The history of Chinese medicine was a contentious one, with many disputes among different medical schools. Its indigenous traditions include the Wen Bing approach, which emerged in the late Ming Dynasty and steered Chinese medicine in a different direction from Korea's over the course of the succeeding Qing Dynasty. One difference is that the Chinese approach focuses on curing disease with what is called "dialectical treatment." Developments in this field were focused on infectious diseases.

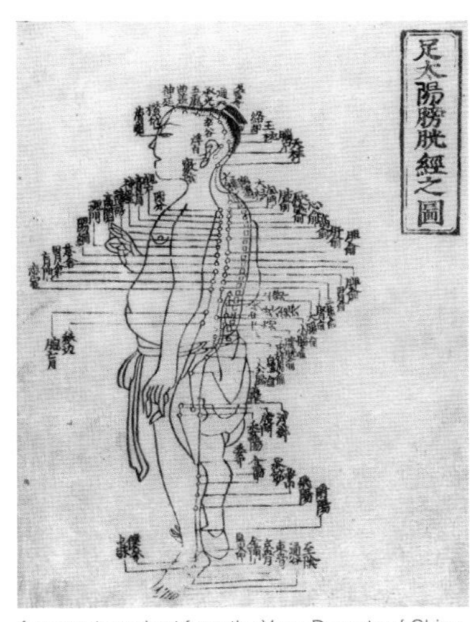

Acupuncture chart from the Yuan Dynasty of China

Starting in the 1950s, the communist government began adopting a three-part system combining Chinese and Western medicine: purely Chinese, purely Western, and a hybrid of the two. Despite its name, what is called traditional Chinese medicine (TCM) today is a modernized form that is considered distinct from traditional Chinese medicine.

Like Korea, Japan was also influenced by Chinese medicine. Unlike Korea, however, Japan lost its institutional system of Oriental medicine after the Meiji Restoration and in its place, individual practitioners of acupuncture and herbal medicine emerged. The herbal treatments from that era are still widely used today; close to 70 percent of physicians have experience prescribing some form. As a result, active clinical research has yielded many useful findings over the years.

With Japan abandoning its official system in the 19th century and China adopting a more pragmatic combination of traditional and Western approaches in the second half of the 20th, Korea has remained the truest to its roots among all traditions of East Asian medicine.

Sasang Medicine

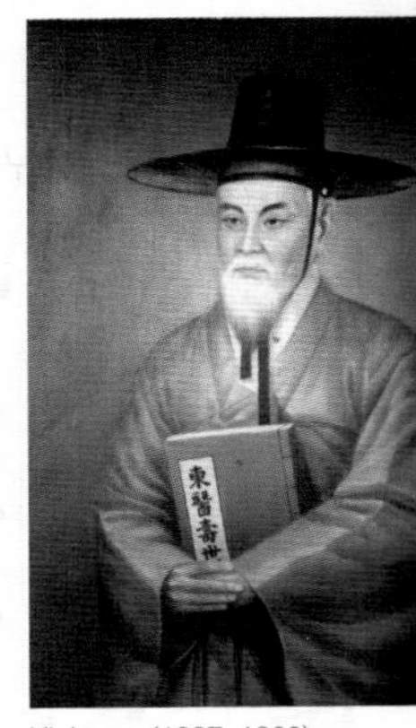
Yi Je-ma (1837–1900)

With a name meaning "four constitutional forms," *sasang* medicine is a unique and creative theoretical approach to treatment. First laid out by Joseon physician Yi Je-ma in his book *Donguisusebowon*, it presented something completely different from the mainstream Korean medicine of the day. It took the four constitutional forms from the "Two Polarities Diagram" in the *I Ching*—*taeyang* (big *yang*), *soyang* (small *yang*), *taeeum* (big *yin*), and *soeum* (small *yin*)—and applied them to the human body to determine the cause of diseases, proper treatment, and ways of maintaining health. Each person was classified as one of the four types based on traits and personality, and suitable methods of treatment were prescribed for each. In other words, constitution was emphasized over symptoms even in treatment; two people with the same ailment but different constitutions would not receive the same treatment.

The central issue in *sasang* medicine was the classification of constitutions. Yi offered different methods for doing this, some associated with appearance (face and body shape), others with personality, and others based on specific symptoms and responses to herbal remedies. Ideally, examinations focused on build: a person's weight might go up or down after marriage or childbirth, and he or she might be affected by factors such as nutrition, exercise, or illness, but innate constitution would not change much. Similarly, because personality can be influenced by learning and habit—and because a person might show his or her true character when forced into extreme circumstances in which a crucial decision must be made—any examination had to be done scrupulously and over several sessions.

Among ways of detecting disease include checking a person's sweat, urine, and feces. For example, a *taeeum* person tends to sweat a lot but feels refreshed afterwards; he or she also drinks a lot of water. A *soeum* person feels more tired after sweating, and does not drink as much water. A *soyang* person who goes for days without bowel movement will experience a feeling of unbearable constriction in the chest, while a *soeum* person under the same circumstances will not feel particularly troubled. A *taeeum* person, in contrast, might have two or three soft bowel movements a day.

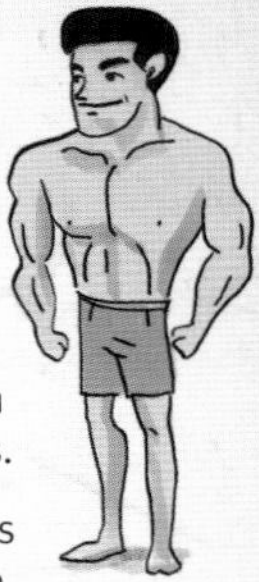

Taeyang: Broad-chested and broad-shouldered. The back of the neck is thick, but the lower back is weak. Weak legs result in shaky posture and the inability to stand or walk for long periods of time. The body is not fleshy and the face is clearly defined, but because this is the rarest of the four types—as ten in every 10,000 people—it can be difficult to distinguish. *Taeyang* people are clever, creative, and masculine, with an active and energetic spirit. They are also skinny, with sharp and glinting eyes.

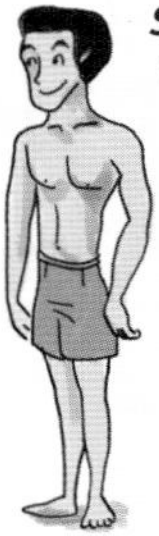

Soyang: Full-chested, with weakly defined buttocks. Women of this type tend to have large breasts. *Soyang* people are active, passionate, and impatient. They have many bright ideas and tend to work well, but also lack perseverance; they often have difficulty finishing what they start and grow easily frustrated. They are often thin, with piercing eyes and a sharp nose. This type is relatively common, representing around 3,000 out of every 10,000 people. The characteristics are usually quite apparent, making *soyang* people fairly easy to spot.

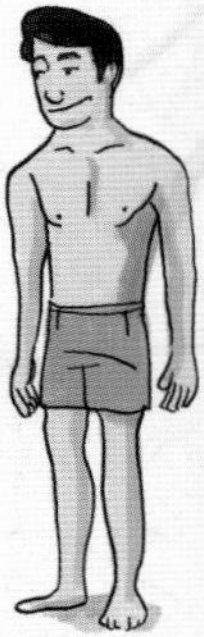

Taeeum: *Taeeum* people have strong backs and a seemingly sturdy posture when standing, but the back of their neck appears relatively weak. Most are strongly built and fleshy, giving them a reliable appearance. Their calmness and quietness make them seem trustworthy, but they do appear impatient at times. They are honest (sometimes to a fault) and persevering; they always finish what they start and may come across as conservative. They can also be devious, lazy, greedy, and complacent. Their body appears clearly defined. Representing 5,000 of every 10,000 people, they are the easiest type to identify.

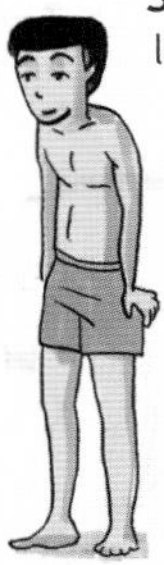

Soeum: *Soeum* people tend to have developed lower bodies, with large buttocks and thick legs. They appear stable when seated, but their waistlines are weak. They often have a neat appearance and small frame, giving them a docile look and a tendency to disappear into the crowd. They are mild-mannered and sedate, affable and social, and nearly always surrounded by people. They are quite meticulous and careful in planning, but they can also be passive and feminine: they dislike getting involved in other people's business, are acutely aware where their interests lie, and are prone to intense jealousy. They generally have thin and frail frames. They represent about 2,000 of every 10,000 people.

Chapter Two

BASIC PRINCIPLES AND PHILOSOPHIES

YIN, YANG, AND THE FIVE ELEMENTS

The theory of *yin* and *yang* and the five elements of wood, fire, earth, metal and water is a philosophical system that developed millennia ago in China. The ancients used the theory to interpret and deduce the nature, changes, and development of every object in nature. Combined with the principles of medicine, it came to represent a basic theoretical approach for explaining the relationship between people and nature and examining medical issues.

Yin and Yang

In the *yin/yang* hypothesis, everything that happens in nature is assigned to one of these two categories. But whichever one it is, it is also understood to contain its opposite; *yin* phenomena have a *yang* side and vice versa. In other words, they are interdependent, existing in a cyclical relationship of flourishing and decay and qualitative change. Combined with the diagnostic and treatment methods of medicine, this system offers a way of understanding the fundamentals of disease by distinguishing the *yin* and *yang* aspects.

The hypothesis has four main parts:

- **Opposition:** The hypothesis holds that all objects have paired and opposing *yin* and *yang* aspects. The sky, for example, is *yang*, while the earth is *yin*; daytime is *yang*, night is *yin*. The material substance of the body is *yin*, while its functional side is *yang*. Viscera, being internal, are *yin*; the surface of the body, being external, is *yang*. There are also the *yin* organs (the five viscera) and *yang* organs (the six bowels).

Model of the human body with meridians and acupuncture points

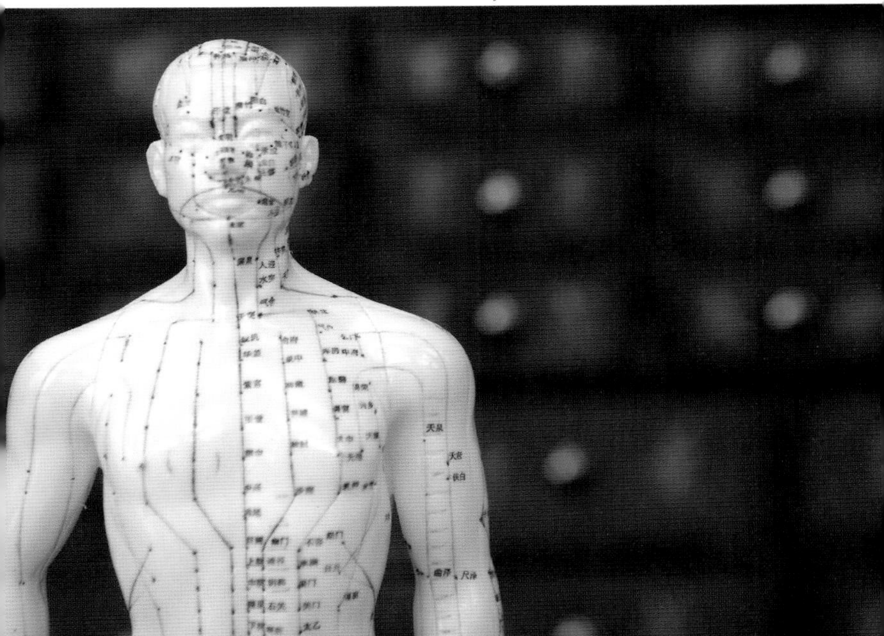

- **Dependence:** *Yin* and *yang* exist in opposition, but in an interdependent opposition, where one cannot exist without the other. In other words, neither *yin* nor *yang* can exist alone. When shining a light on an object, the illuminated side is its *yang*, while the shadow is its *yin*. Shade cannot exist without the sun; sunny places cannot exist without shade. As mentioned before, the body's functions are seen as *yang* and its substance as *yin*; there can be no function without substance and no substance without function.
- **Flourishing and Decay:** When describing the relationship between *yin* and *yang* as oppositional and interdependent, this also means that the relationship is not static or unchanging. Indeed, it is constantly going through a process of extinction and growth like the changing of the seasons. As winter gives way to spring and summer, there is a process of *yin* decaying and *yang* flourishing as the weather goes from cold to warm. Similarly, the period from

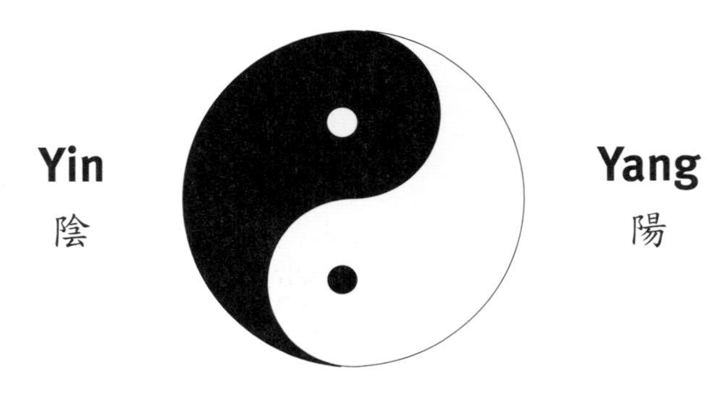

summer through fall and on to winter is one of *yang* decaying and *yin* flourishing as the weather goes from warm to cold. While the body's functions are viewed as *yang*, their activity depends on the consumption of *yin* nutrients. Metabolizing nutrients requires a certain amount of energy, and when the mutual ebb and flow of the two aspects loses balance, illness is the result.

- **Transformation:** Objects may start as either *yin* [illegible] but once they reach a certain stage in their developme[illegible] [illegible]ansform into their opposite. Thus *yin* becomes *yang* and [illegible] [illegible]mes *yin*.

The Five Elements

From the perspective of natural science, the hypothesis of the five elements might seem like a kind of atomic theory. This theory holds that all things in the universe originate with the movement and changes of five materials: wood, fire, earth, metal, and water. Called the "five elements," they are forever moving and changing in interlocking patterns of activity and suppression. When applied to medicine, this approach offers a way not just to explain the physiology and pathology of the human body, but also its relationship with the outside world. It also supplies an important theoretical underpinning for diagnosis and treatment.

The major components of the hypothesis include:

- **Symbiosis:** The "bio" part of this word—"life"—includes the ideas of activity and encouragement. The elements follow a set sequence: wood encourages fire, fire encourages earth, earth encourages metal, metal encourages water, and water encourages wood. Thus trees are understood to grow from water because water encourages wood; the water represents the kidneys, the wood the liver. The kidneys are the mother of the liver, so both exist in a kind of mother-and-child relationship.

- **Suppression:** Suppression, or exhaustion, also follows a set sequence in which an element affects the one that is two places after it: wood suppresses earth, earth suppresses water, water suppresses fire, fire suppresses metal, and metal suppresses wood. In the relationship of fire suppressing metal, for example, metal is understood to be the lungs and fire the heart. When a person has intense fire energy in his or her heart, he or she risks serious damage to the lungs since fire is capable of melting metal.

- **Vanquishing:** This is a process of excessive suppression in which one element takes advantage of another's weakness to invade it. For example, wood is typically supposed to suppress earth, but if a person's earth energy is too weak, then the wood's suppression grows too intense and disrupts normal balance.

- **Contempt:** This involves believing too much in one's own strength and despising or insulting weakness. When earth energy is too strong, for example, wood energy can no longer suppress it. Instead, the reverse happens: earth energy suppresses wood energy.

Under normal circumstances, the first two of these, symbiosis and suppression, are closely connected. This is essential if the body is to remain healthy: growth cannot happen without encouragement, and the normal processes of change and development cannot happen without suppression. The latter two, vanquishing and contempt, are abnormal processes in the development and changing of objects and can result in pathological conditions.

DIAGRAM OF THE FIVE ELEMENTS

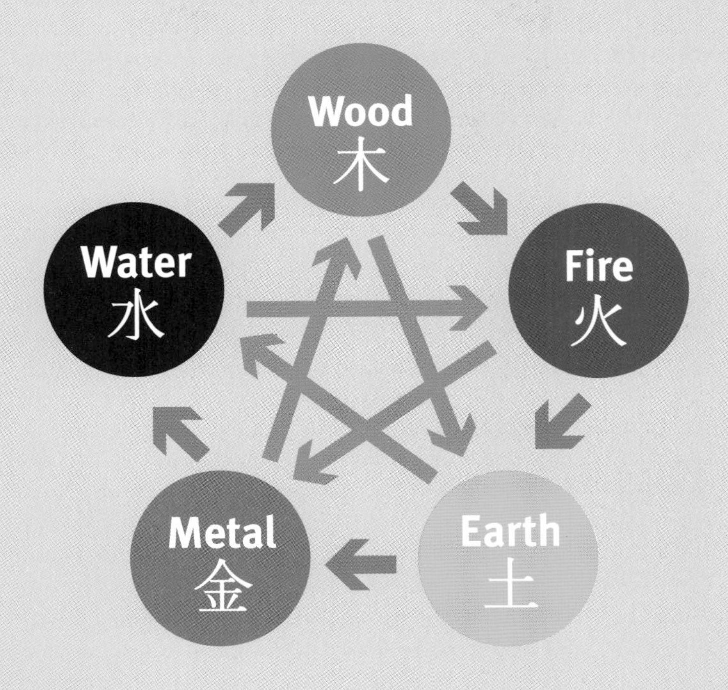

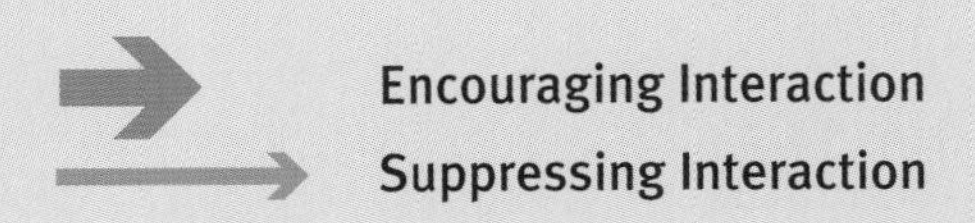

THE 'WHOLE BODY' CONCEPT

In Korean traditional medicine, the body is fundamentally understood as an integrated whole, inside and out, with two corresponding *yin* and *yang* elements. Practitioners have observed its upper and lower portions, or interior and exterior; internal organs are divided into viscera and bowels and the basic elements of the body into energy and blood. In functional terms, the whole is understood through the movements of internal correspondence and integration between its elements: the physiological order arises from the decay and flourishing of *yin* and *yang*, and from changes in energy and blood. When this system is disrupted, disease follows. In other words, the different parts of the body are not separate but connected and corresponding, with physiological and pathological phenomena resulting from their interactions.

A similar perspective applies to the relationship between people and their environment. Since people live their lives within nature, the conditions of nature are the conditions of human survival, and thus changes in nature's conditions will impact the human body. People rely on nature to keep them alive, and can continue to grow as they adapt to the changing seasons. But once natural circumstances deviate from their rules, the result is disorder in the body's ability to adjust normally. The normal order between humans and their environment breaks down, and disease is the result.

In Korean traditional medicine, the phenomena of nature and body, for all their differences, are understood to follow common rules. A good explanation for this can be found in the *Huangdi Neijing* (Inner Canon of Huangdi), a classic of Oriental medicine. "Illness is healed in the morning, for it is the time of day that is like spring, when *yang* energy is alive and the energy of disease is weakening," it reads. "Midday is like summer, when *yang* energy is at its fullest. The body's energy is at its strongest and the disease's energy is at its weakest. Evening is like fall, when *yang* energy is weakening and the disease's energy is beginning to grow; thus, our illness gradually worsens. And the night is like winter: our *yang* energy is dormant and the disease's energy is flourishing, so our illness is at its worst."

Meridians, Energy, and Blood

Meridians

Meridians (*gyeongnak* in Korean) are the main channels by which energy, blood, and essence travel through the body. They spread to every part of the body in a network of interconnecting pathways. They link organs and tissues through characteristic routes that turn the body into one organic whole. They identify the relationships and influence between systems, reflect the body's physiological phenomena and pathology, and regulate the cycle of energy and blood throughout the body. In short, meridians are the body's

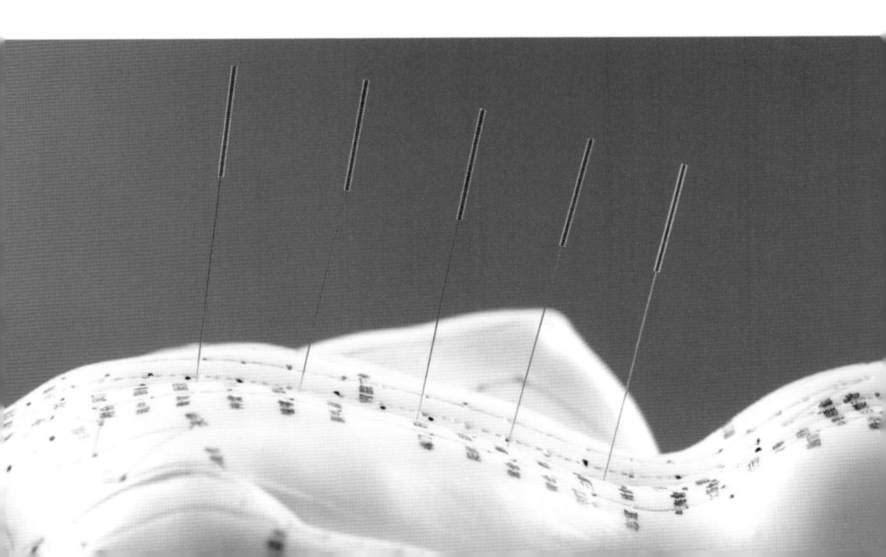

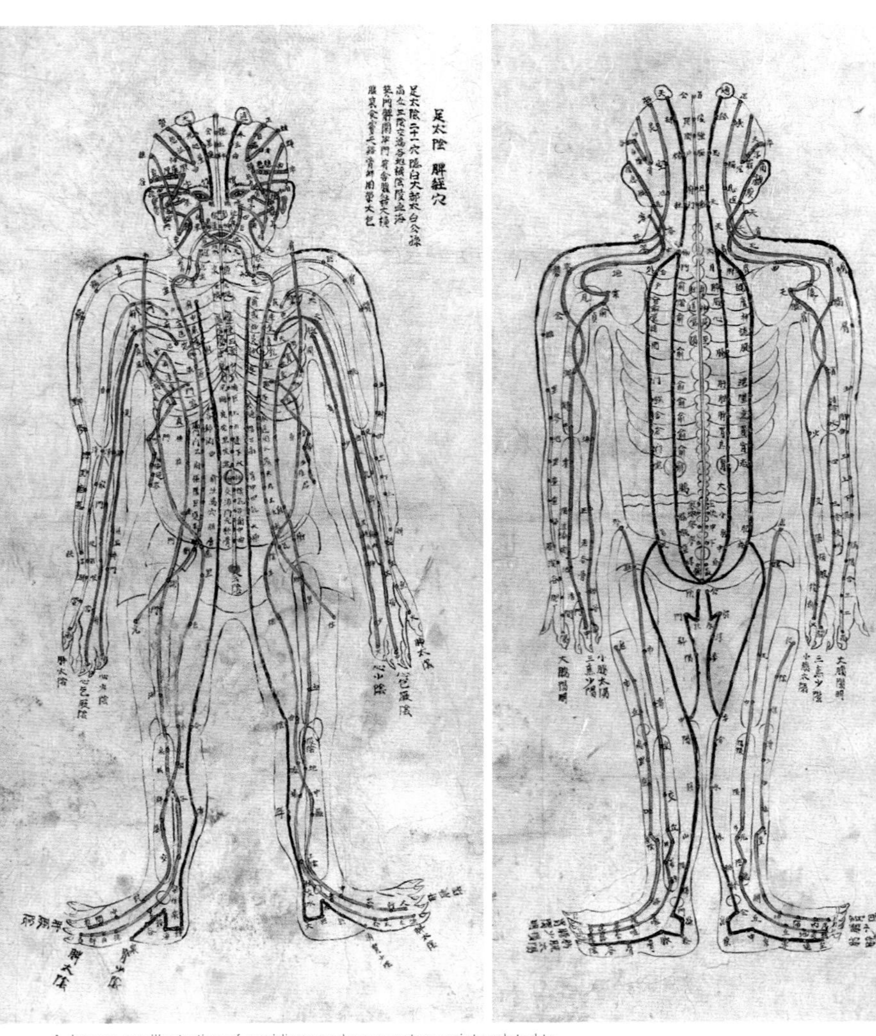

A Joseon-era illustration of meridians and acupuncture points related to the circulatory system and flow of energy channels for connection, reaction, and regulation.

The body depends on supplies of energy and blood to keep functioning normally, and through meridians, they are transported throughout the body to do what they need to. The energy, blood, and essence stemming from the things people eat can thus reach every part of the body. But the meridians are not merely pathways for essence; they also allow the circulation of energy to protect against disease-causing pathogens outside.

Whenever the functioning of internal organs is disrupted by pathogens or a kind of disease results, a reaction in the corresponding area of a body's meridians occurs. A disease of the intestines, for example, elicits a reaction on part of the body's surface because of meridian connections. This also means that diseases of the intestines can be examined by observing or pressing on these parts.

Acupuncture is used to treat diseases by way of meridians that pass over or control areas where the pathogens are located. A practitioner can treat a condition not only by stimulating the affected area, but also by stimulating distant, linked meridians.

The two types of meridians are channels and collaterals. Channels are the main pathways, typically circulating deeply through parts of the body through clearly defined pathways. Collaterals are branches of these channels that link to different parts of the body in a kind of meshwork patterns. The channels can be divided into two types: 12 "regular meridians" and eight "extraordinary meridians." The 12 regular meridians are subdivided into "hand" and "foot" depending on the location of the meridian routes, as well as *yin* and *yang* types, and then assigned to each of the five viscera and six bowels, for a total of 12 names. The eight extraordinary meridians correspond to these 12 regular meridians. Collaterals are generally horizontally distributed as they link channels. Their purpose is to support the circulation of energy, blood, and nutrients in areas of the body that the channels do not reach.

Energy and Blood

The term "energy" (*gi* in Korean, *qi* in Chinese) is used in a very broad sense in Korean traditional medicine. In its simplest terms, energy is anything capable of causing action. All things in the universe arise and disappear through the changing movements of energy. In the human body, energy is understood as the activity of life. Lack of energy in the body would mean all physical and mental activities would cease, leaving behind nothing but form. The origins of energy in the body lie in the substances produced through respiration in the lungs and digestion of food in the stomach.

The five principal types of energy in the body are:

- **Impulsion:** Physical growth, the functions of organs and meridians, blood circulation, and the transport of nutrients all take place through energy impulsion.

- **Warmth:** Adjustments of energy are what allow people to maintain normal body temperature. When this warming action is not properly working, the ability to regulate body temperature is lost, resulting in symptoms like chills and coldness in the limbs.

- **Control:** The controlling action of energy keeps blood from leaking outside its vessels. It also ensures that sweat and urine are released normally.

- **Defense:** Energy protects the skin from external pathogens. When it weakens, the body cannot defend itself and pathogens intrude to cause disease and bring a toxic energy that triggers resistance.

- **Transformation:** This function is related to the organs and allows the transformation of energy, blood, and essence.

Blood is the *yin* to energy's *yang*. Where energy is mainly concerned with functions, blood is a nutrient and important fuel for the body's manifestations. Food that has been converted into "essence" by the actions of the stomach enters the heart by the actions of the lungs. Through the impulsion actions of the heart and energy, it circulates through the body's meridians.

This cycling takes it both inside to the five viscera and six bowels, and outside to the skin, muscles, and bones to supply nutrients wherever needed. All organs—the skin, hair, the meridians of muscles and bone, and the intestines—receive their nutrients through the blood. Blood also forms the physical basis of mental activity. The mind, practitioners of Korean traditional medicine have held, is clear only if the body has sufficient energy and blood.

Internal Organs: The Five Viscera and Six Bowels

The "internal organs" as described by Korean traditional medicine do not conform exactly to the anatomical organs of Western medicine. In Korean traditional medicine, organs are categorized by functional similarity into a kind of systematic framework. In keeping with the theory of *yin*, *yang*, and the five elements, they form a functional system that encompasses all of the different actions of the body. There are viscera (*yin*) and bowels (*yang*), with each of the viscera assigned one of the five elements. *Gan*, which is one of the five viscera, is

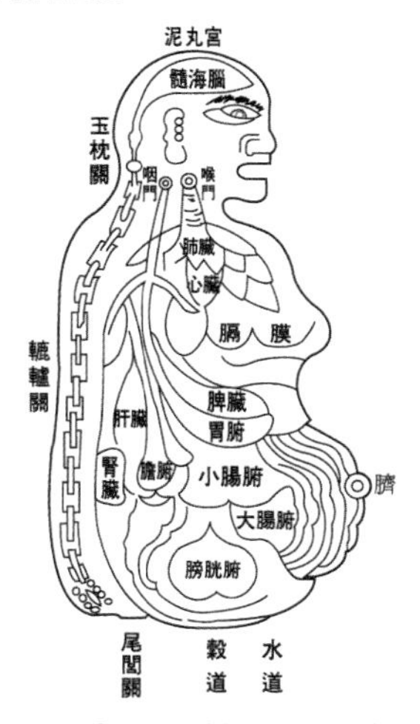

Diagram of the viscera and bowls from the *Donguibogam*

commonly translated as "liver," but this is not just the organ taught in an anatomy class. Rather, the organ directs blood, aids digestion, helps energy and blood flow throughout the body, and controls anger and thought, with its state reflected in the fingernails and muscles. In other words, the organ is more of a "conceptual" liver within a more general functional system.

The five viscera are *gan* (liver), *sim* (heart), *bi* (spleen), *pye* (lungs), and *sin* (kidneys). They guard the essential forces of the body—*yin* and *yang*, energy and blood—along with a person's psychological and emotional state. The six bowels are the *dam* (gall bladder), *sojang* (small intestine), *wi* (stomach), *daejang* (large intestine), *banggwang* (bladder), and *samcho* (the "three burners"). They are responsible for digesting and absorbing the food and water taken in from nature and turning them into vital energy, while eliminating unnecessary waste matter from the body.

When arranged according to the five elements, the five viscera and six bowels form the following functional pairs:

- ***Gan/dam:*** The liver stores blood, aids digestion, and helps energy and blood flow throughout the body. It also controls muscles, and its characteristics are shown in the fingernails. Its control extends to the eyes, and the liver forms a pair with the *dam* (gall bladder).

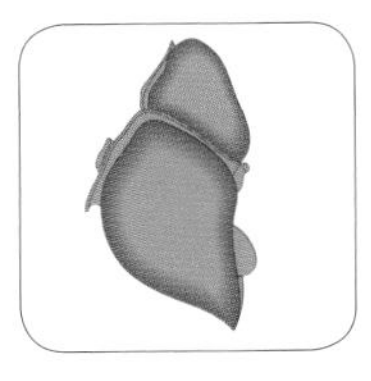

- ***Sim/sojang:*** The heart controls the blood, along with a person's mind and consciousness. Its state can be determined by looking at the tongue, and its bowel counterpart is the *sojang*(small intestine).

- ***Bi/wi:*** The spleen digests food and converts it to essential energy. Its bowel counterpart is *wi* (stomach). The

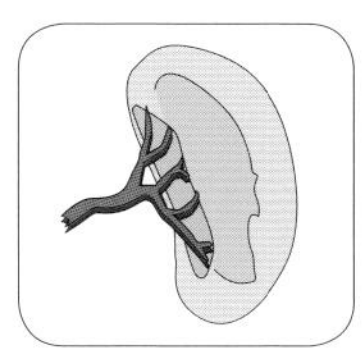

spleen ensures that blood does not leak from blood vessels. When the spleen is not working properly, bruising or hemorrhage can result. Its characteristics are often seen in the limbs, mouth, and lips.

- ***Pye/daejang:*** The lungs control energy and are closely linked to breathing. They are also crucial to fluid metabolism, spreading fluid throughout the body and influencing excretion. They control the skin, and their condition can be observed through the nose. Their bowel counterpart is the *daejang* (large intestine).

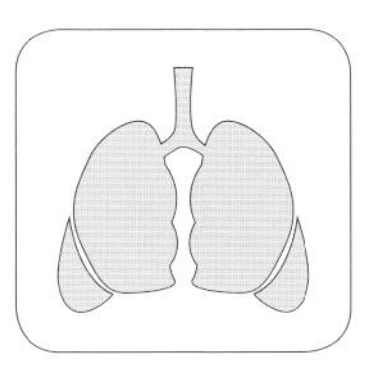

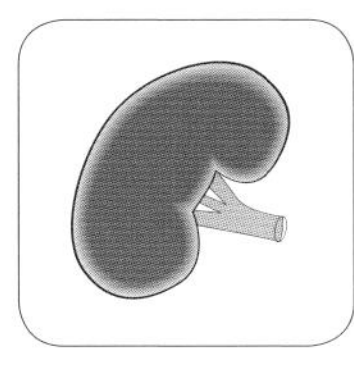

- ***Sin/banggwang:*** The kidneys control the body's innate vital energy, along with physical growth, development, and reproduction. They are involved in fluid metabolism, and their state can be seen in the ears. They also affect bones and participate in marrow formation. Their bowel counterpart is the *banggwang* (bladder).

- ***Samcho:*** Included among the six bowels is a kind of "intangible organ" that lacks a concrete shape and exists only in its functions. There is an "upper burner," "middle burner," and "lower burner," depending on the part of the body. The upper burner encompasses the heart and lungs, the middle burner the stomach and liver, and the lower burner the kidneys, large and small intestines, and bladder. Together, they control the transforming actions of the body (the functions of each organ through the actions of energy and blood) and provide channels for fluid flow.

3 Chapter Three

DIAGNOSIS: THE FOUR METHODS

The principles of Korean traditional medicine require an assessment of eight symptoms grouped into four pairs: cold/hot, deficiency/sufficiency, large/small, and *yin/yang*. Even if a patient exhibits symptoms usually associated with a known disorder, a doctor of Korean traditional medicine makes a diagnosis in accordance with symptom groupings and prescribes the appropriate treatment. Also important is detection of any negative energy entering a patient's body, and to consider characteristics of the patient's physique, face type, personality, and lifestyle to determine the most effective treatment for each individual.

Korean traditional medicine normally applies four methods of diagnosis: visual examination, listening/smelling, inquiry, and palpation. These basic ways are how a physician examines the patient and understands his or her ailment. The first method, visual examination, is observing the patient's condition with the eyes. In listening/smelling, the sounds and odors of the body are examined. Inquiry involves asking the patient about how the disease began and how it has changed, along with any existing symptoms. Finally, palpation mainly involves taking the pulse and checking parts of the body by touch. When using these methods, the physician must not put too much emphasis on any one of them; an accurate diagnosis depends on a comprehensive analysis that uses information from all four.

Visual Examination

Visual examination is the most basic diagnostic approach. The physician must use his or her eyes to examine the patient, both in general and for particular parts of the body, to understand the characteristics and condition of the ailment. In the mental examination, the physician examines different areas—general

A foreign patient has her pulse taken at a Korean traditoinal medicine clinic.

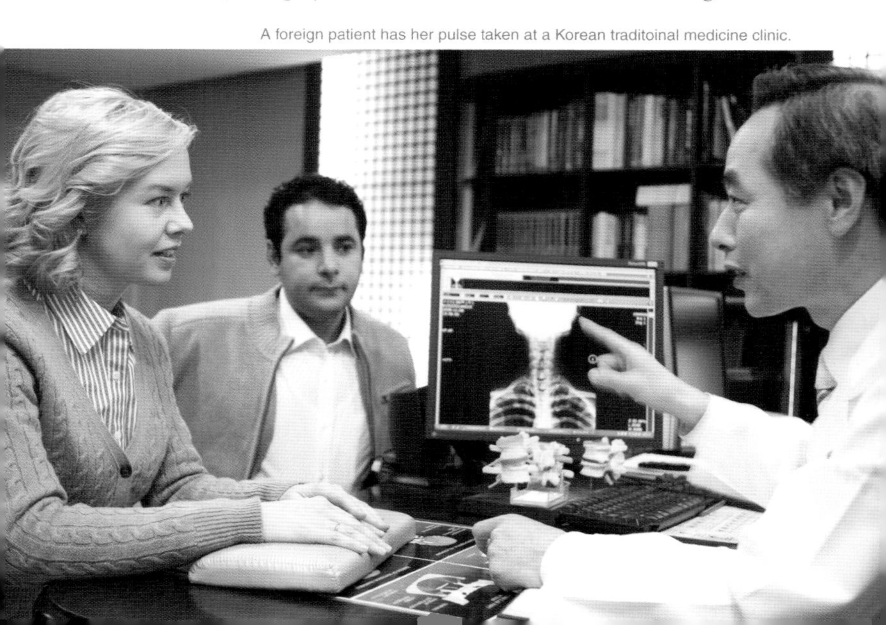

soundness of mind, the glimmer in the patient's eye, clarity of language and response—for diagnosis and predict whether it will get better or worse.

Another examination is the physical examination, in which the physician diagnoses disease by looking at the patient's development and movement. In particular, he examines whether the body is too fat or thin; checks for any paralysis, twitching, shuddering, or other strange movement; and searches for structural issues with the body such as shrinkage or twisting.

Because the color and luster of the face are closely related to the presence or absence of energy and blood in the body, another part of the examination is observation of facial coloring. Typically, an Asian patient has a slightly yellow cast to the skin, with a touch of red coloring and slight shine, but these colors change when disease is present. A person with fever will have a reddened complexion, while someone who is very weak will appear pale. In addition to the face, the physician also has to examine the rest of the patient's skin to look for mottling or redness and assess the overall condition.

The last and most crucial part of the diagnosis is examination of the tongue. This diagnosis holds great meaning in Korean traditional medicine. The shape and color of the organ are understood to reflect the flourishing or weakening of energy and blood in the body, and signaling if the patient will

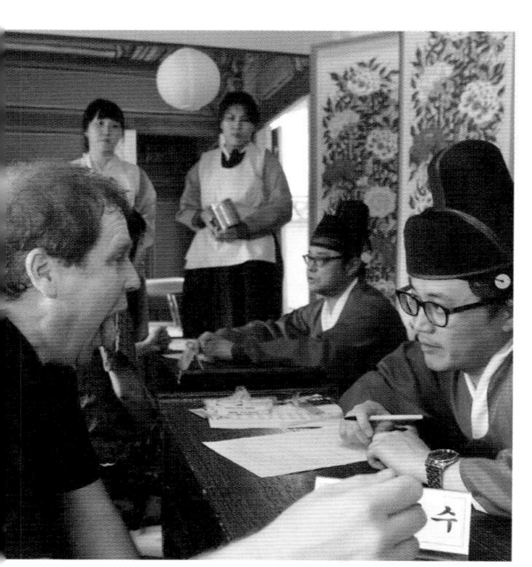

A foreign visitor has his tongue examined in a reenactment of a Joseon royal medicine procedure.

improve or get worse, whether the ailment is hot or cold, and whether the disease has strong or weak energy. The inspection consists of two parts: observing the body of the tongue and looking at its coating.

The body of the tongue can say a mouthful (so to speak). A large, swollen tongue strongly suggests weakness of bodily energy, or possibly edema. A thin and frail tongue, in contrast, suggests lack of nutrients or a wasting disease. A tongue that is too darkly red indicates inflammation, while a purple shade means that blood is leaking somewhere in the body. If the tongue's movement is not smooth or if signs of paralysis are present, this often suggests a problem with the central nervous system. Too much shaking often means high fever or an overactive thyroid.

Most people have a thin white coating on their tongue. The problem occurs when the coat is too thick; this means the disease's energy is highly active and the condition is likely to get worse. The color also shares information about the body's condition. Yellow typically indicates fever and often occurs in the presence of an inflammatory infection. A dark, blackish coating indicates acuteness and abundance of disease energy, and is often present when the patient is suffering from an acute suppurating infection such as peritonitis, cholecystitis, or septicemia.

Listening/Smelling

In the listening/smelling part of the diagnosis, the physician listens to the patient's voice and speech, breathing, coughing, and other sounds of the body and checks the scents of his or her secretions and excretions, and other odors.

The first part of this method is listening to the patient's pronunciation, language, and breathing to better understand the ailment. Changes in speech and breathing are a direct indication of changes in the disease; any problems in speaking or answering questions are typically associated with problems of the mind and consciousness. A person with faint, halting speech who is difficult to understand and has short breath and panting is likely to have impaired lung function; a thick voice and coarse breathing are likely signs of a kind of pathogen. If the patient's words make no sense (non-sequiturs or bizarre answers), this is considered a sign of problems with heart function, an organ that governs the mind. Coughing and hiccups also provide important information for diagnosing changes in disease.

The physician can gain a better understanding of a condition by smelling the patient's breath and body odors, as well as various excrement. Bad breath indicates gastric fever and could provide a vital clue in diagnosing ailments of the gastrointestinal tract. Just as the characteristic body odor from serious and chronic diabetes comes from an increase in ketonic acid, the smells of a body can provide a doctor of Korean traditional medicine with a way of diagnosing disease. The concentration and odor of excretions such as phlegm, urine, feces, and sweat may be caused by heat toxins, while watery, odorless excretions indicate lack of energy.

INQUIRY

Inquiry is an important part of the diagnostic process; many physicians over the years say it is the single most important step. Asking a patient directly about his or her condition can help the physician not only understand more about how the disease started and developed, but also past experiences, family history, and social factors that can help predict changes in the disease and set a treatment. While the patient's symptoms are obviously important,

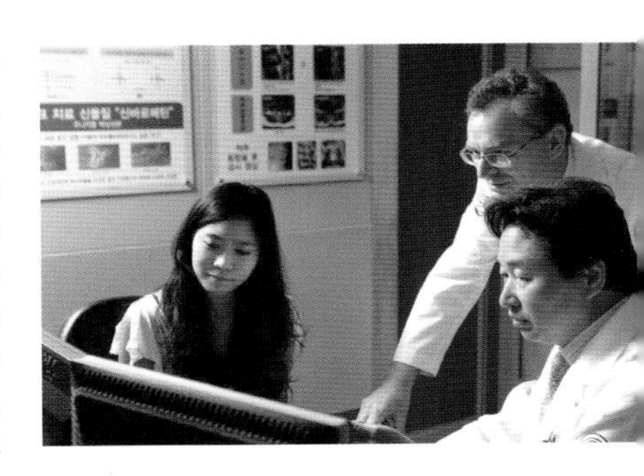

understanding of the body's normal condition allows for a more sophisticated approach to treating it. But because this method depends on subjective ratings from the patient, the physician must also supplement it with the more objective methods of visual examination, listening/smelling, and palpation to make a more accurate diagnosis.

Through inquiry, a physician can determine:

- whether the patient is suffering from fever or chills and if they are appearing separately or together.
- whether the patient is sweating. Sweat is seen as a product of the body's essence, and any abnormalities in sweat indicate problems with that essence. A person who sweats excessively during the day or at the slightest physical activity often suffers from weakness of *yang* energy; someone who sweats heavily while sleeping at night is likely to have weak *yin* energy.
- condition of urine and feces. These excrements are the remnants of food digested and absorbed by the body, which means they also provide the most direct way of observing the condition of the gastrointestinal tract and kidney function. Chronic diarrhea or constipation, frequent urination (especially at night), and difficulty controlling the bladder can be good ways of determining the body's normal condition. Constipation, for example, is seen as indicating a high level of heat in the body: essence is being consumed, resulting in a harder stool. This could also mean that the body is not excreting properly because of

weaker peristalsis in the intestines. In the first case, treatment involves supplementing essence and lowering body heat. In the second, the intent is to improve gastrointestinal tract function so peristalsis can occur normally.

- appetite, including whether the patient experiences thirst and hunger and how digestion is.
- condition of the chest and abdomen, including chest pains, constriction, and stomach pain.
- sleep patterns. In Korean traditional medicine, sleep patterns are seen as connected to the heart, which governs the mind, and the liver, which controls the blood. Difficulty falling asleep, the inability to sleep deeply, and certain types of dreams might indicate lack of blood in the heart or liver.
- general condition of the head and body. Typically, the patient will be asked about headaches, dizziness, heat in the head, pain in different parts of the body, lumps, and other problems.
- pre-existing conditions. The physician will often ask about past illnesses and their treatment, as well as any restrictions on medicine.

PALPATION

In palpation, the physician feels parts of the patient's body with his hand to understand more about the patient's condition. This includes pulse-taking, along with a more general examination of the body.

When taking a pulse, the physician looks at both its condition and quality. He or she conducts the examination by pressing the tips of the index, middle, and ring finger against the inside of the patient's wrist and moving them, in turn, toward the part near the

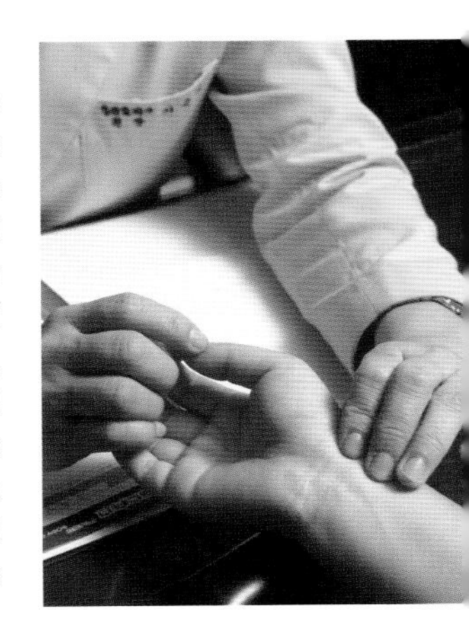

thumb where the radial artery can be felt. The radial styloid process is called *gwan* while the areas in front of and behind it are *chon* and *cheok*. The physician checks pulse for each of these three parts, applying and releasing slight pressure on the fingers. He or she measures the number and strength of beats in a single breath, as well as the size, duration, smoothness or coarseness, and uniformity. Taking the pulse allows diagnosis of the patient's condition and ailments, a decision on a treatment approach, and judgement of a treatment's appropriateness based on the pulse's state before and after.

The palpation examination also includes feeling the abdomen with the finger or palm to check for abnormalities, locate pathogens, and determine how the disease has progressed. When liver energy is stagnant, for example, the patient will report a painful feeling of pressure in both sets of ribs when the physician presses against the eyes. Weak spirit energy is associated with a strong pulse around the navel. Other characteristic abdominal pains make palpation one of the most important clinical methods of diagnosis (along with pulse-checking and inspection of the tongue) in Korean traditional medicine.

Specific meridians are associated with specific organs, and certain acupoints represent the condition of those meridians; for example, the *baesu* point for the upper back and the *bongmo* point for the stomach. By pressing on these points, the condition of the corresponding organ can be assessed.

The last part of palpation is examination of the skin, especially its coolness and heat, luster, and dryness. The physician will also feel for coolness and warmth in the arms and legs.

Chapter Four

METHODS OF TREATMENT

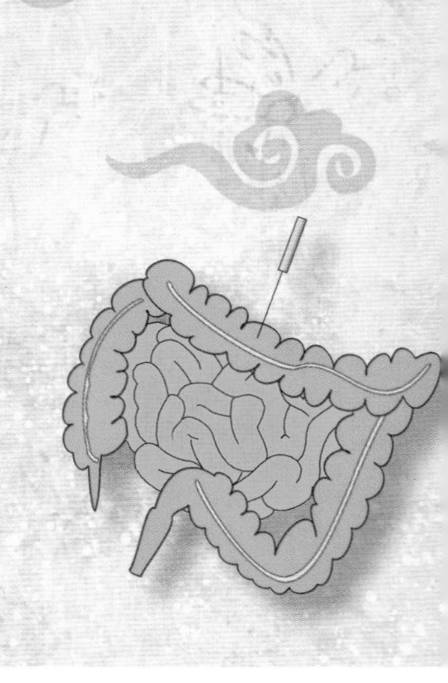

In its simplest terms, Korean traditional medicine follows a treatment principle called *bujeonggeosa*, which seeks to dispel evil energies by supporting proper functioning of the body's *qi*, or energy. Diseases are generally blamed on the weakening of right energy; the body's resistance is degraded, leaving it unable to defend itself against disease-causing bad energy from outside. Because of this, the strengthening of right energy is a major part of the cure. When a cold virus invades the body, a person with strong resistance will not get ill, but someone with a weak body and low resistance will get sick by even the most minor of pathogens. This means that treatment is not just about eliminating bad energy from outside, but also about strengthening right energy within.

Another important principle is that treatment should consider the patient's constitution. Instead of solely focusing on symptoms, treatment varies from one individual to the next; the same set of symptoms might be treated in very different ways. Two people might eat the same food, yet only one of them will experience indigestion, headache, or vomiting. The same is true for medicine; it can serve as a tonic with positive effects in one person but cause negative side effects in another.

Acupuncture, moxibustion, and herbal medicine are the most popular applications of Korean traditional medicine, which represent a synthesis of research in the medical and natural sciences along with roots in Eastern philosophy. Adherents of Korean traditional medicine are known to recommend the use of acupuncture first, moxibustion second, and herbal medicine third. These three practices, which form the most effective applications of Korean traditional medicine, are prescribed separately and in combination for medical treatment, depending on a particular disorder and a patient's physical condition.

In Korean traditional medicine, prescriptions must be prepared with the utmost precision to optimize their remedial effects.

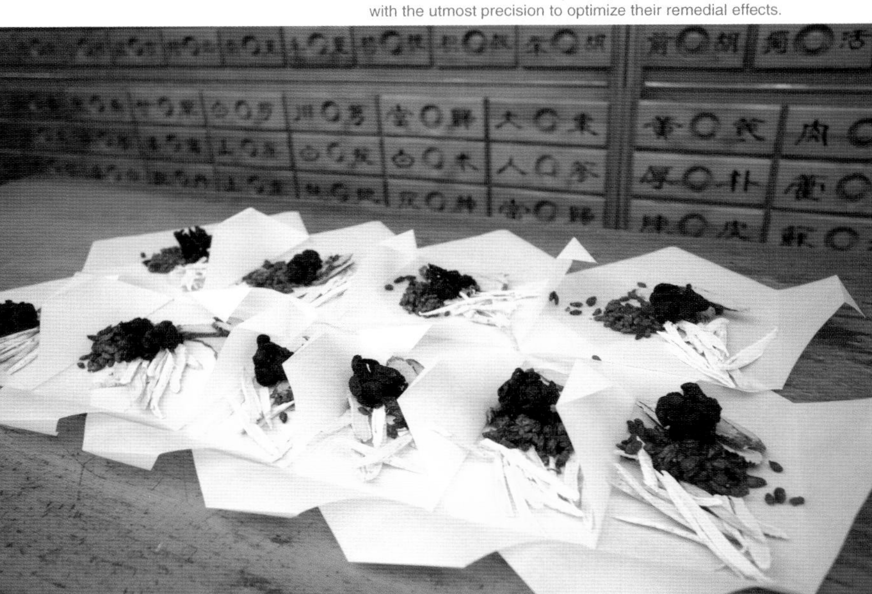

ACUPUNCTURE

Principles and Characteristics

To properly understand acupuncture, familiarity with its principles of meridians and acupuncture points is needed. Within the body is an energy-flow system that regulates organ function from the head to the feet, and laterally from the chest area to the arms. These channels, along which energy flows through the body, are known as meridians. Acupuncture points are specified areas for stimulation, and 365 such points are located all over the body. When a person becomes ill and regular energy flow along the meridians is interrupted, acupuncture can remedy an illness or restore physical condition back to normal.

In Korean acupuncture, needles made from refined metals such as gold, silver, and platinum are inserted into the skin to stimulate internal tissue, or can be placed on the skin for surface stimulation.

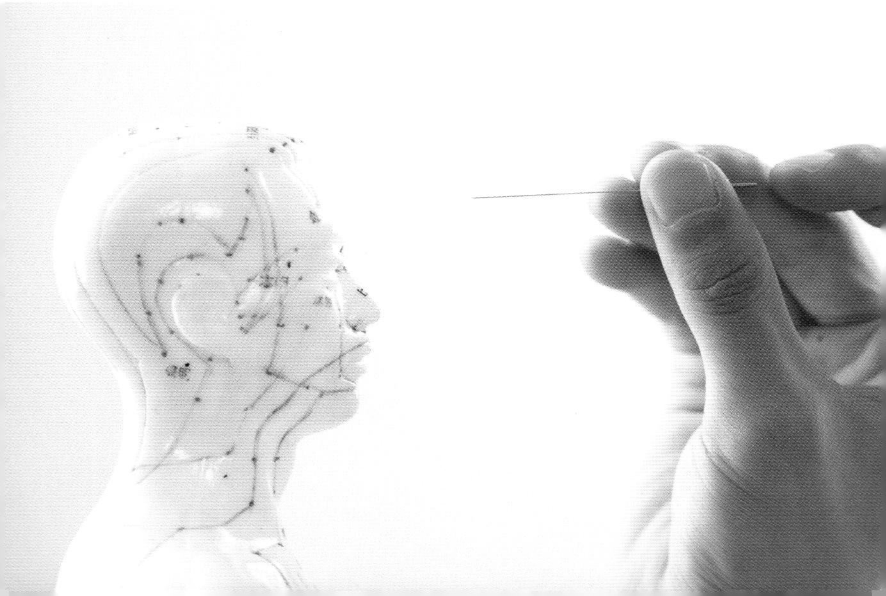

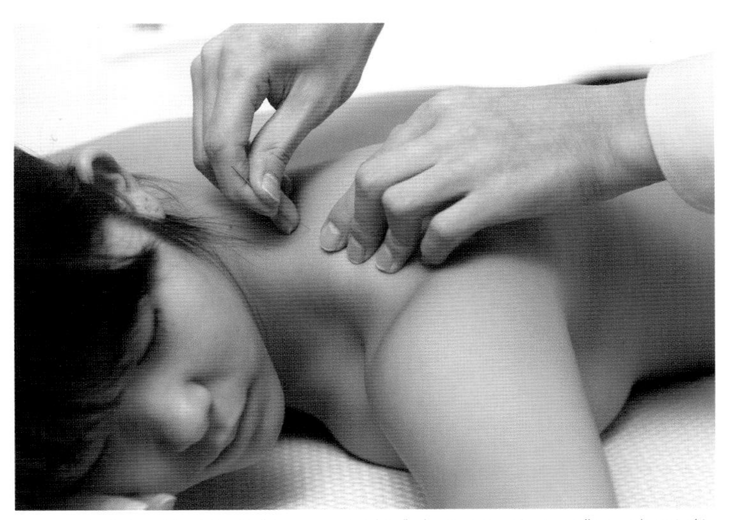

The human body has 365 "acupuncture points," where acupuncture needles are inserted to stimulate the body's energy.

Based on an overall examination and diagnosis, the physician will insert needles into the patient's acupuncture points that are considered conducive to treating a particular ailment. During the insertion, the patient will assume various positions including lying on his or her back, front or side, or sitting in a chair, either upright, leaning to one side, or facing forward with both hands under the chin.

The patient's position and acupuncture points are determined by the treatment methods deemed to be the most effective to remedy the problem. The treatment is often focused around the afflicted area of the body, but can also target seemingly unaffected areas not clearly associated with the disorder. Restoration of the body's proper energy flow is all-important. Depending on the ailment, periodic treatment might be necessary or acupuncture can be combined with physical therapy and the prescription of herbal medicine.

Acupuncture is effective in a wide range of situations, including the treatment of disease, diagnosis of physical disorders, and as a remedial and preventative measure related to fields such as internal medicine, gynecology, pediatrics, psychiatry, surgery, ophthalmology, otorhinolaryngology, and dermatology. Moreover, acupuncture can take effect relatively quickly, is highly effective and economical, and its simple procedures are relatively pain-free and without side effects.

To optimize the efficacy of acupuncture, practitioners of Korean traditional medicine must consider four basic questions. The first is whether to treat the disease or the patient; second is if the treatment should be topical or holistic; third is whether the treatment should focus on the root of the problem or relieve the symptoms; and fourth, whether to strengthen a deficiency or eliminate negative energy. Selection of the proper needles and acupuncture points are also essential based on a patient's specific situation. The most common needles are as fine as a strand of hair and can be inserted with little discomfort. At times, an inserted needle is tapped like a thin nail or twirled to stimulate a wider area. Certain methods involve applying ceramic pieces onto the skin, heating a needle prior to insertion, or inserting a needle and then withdrawing it to extract a small amount of blood.

Korean Forms

Traditional medicine practices unique to Korea include *sa-am* acupuncture, constitutional acupuncture, single-needle acupuncture, and medicinal acupuncture. *Sa-am* is unique in that physical ailments are treated with the insertion of needles exclusively into areas of the arm below the elbow and those of the leg below the knee. In this treatment, inserted needles are manipulated by hand to influence energy flow and diagnose the patient's specific condition. This method is also popular for its ability to provide quick relief.

Constitutional acupuncture is based on a system that categorizes physical constitution into four types: *taeyang*, *taeeum*, *soyang* and *soeum*. In this case, the treatment method is determined by an individual's constitution type as well as the related disorder. Single-needle acupuncture uses the insertion of only one needle into a designated acupuncture point.

Under herbal acupuncture, the treatment includes the insertion of needles and injection of herbal medicine. The prescribed herbal medicine is made into a form that can be applied by syringe and then injected into acupuncture points where needles are also inserted. This combined treatment, which helps to produce immediate benefits for a variety of health problems, has gained wide acceptance in Korea.

A variety of needles are used in acupuncture according to the individual and physical problem.

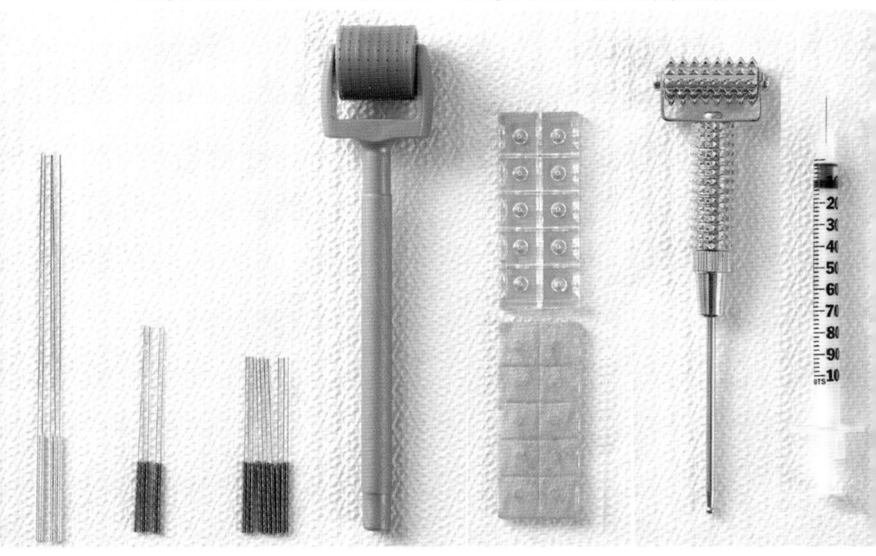

A Cure for Smoking?

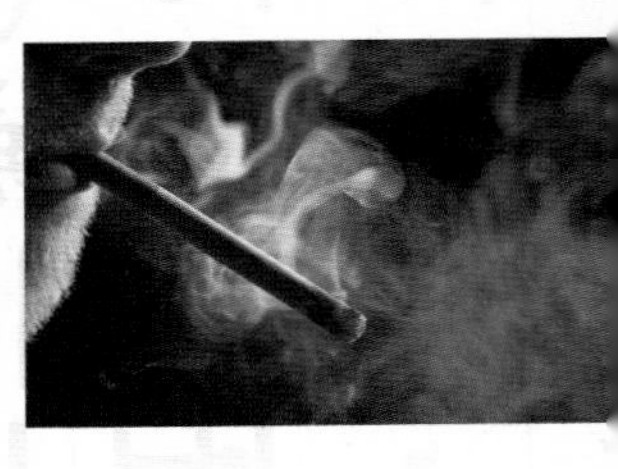

One major application of acupuncture is helping a smoker kick the habit. This kind of acupuncture is different from the typical form, in which long, slender needles are inserted into points all over the body. To overcome smoking, only the ears are treated. The idea behind this new ear treatment is that the organ's shape resembles a fetus in its mother's womb. This is known to be highly effective in other forms of treatment as well, including promoting and suppressing appetite, improving sleeping patterns, and helping to gain strength and achieve better metabolic function. More recently, the method has been adopted for treating obesity and alcohol consumption.

The points selected for treatment represent the course of the cigarette smoke as it moves through the body: the mouth, inner and outer nose, throat, bronchial tubes, lungs, "spirit gate," and internal secretions. The needles are roughly a millimeter long and shaped like small tacks. Once inserted, they are covered with flesh-colored tape and kept on the body throughout the day. The patient is told to apply pressure whenever the urge to smoke arises.

A patient receives treatment in one ear and then the other at intervals of roughly every three days or about twice a week. Around three to four weeks are needed for a patient to quit smoking, though the time period can vary from one person to the next. A person undergoing treatment will have less of an urge to smoke, and cigarettes taste different when he or she decides to indulge. Cigarettes go from being pleasurable to inhale to unpleasant and tasteless, like smoking rolls of paper. People whose response is especially strong will feel nauseated when they smoke, with a sore throat and heavy feeling in the head.

These changes are an important starting point in developing the willpower to quit and staying away from cigarettes for good. But what about someone who cannot say no when offered a cigarette, no matter how unpleasant it tastes? They could adapt to the new sensation—they might reduce the amount they smoke—but cannot quit completely.

Physicians of Korean traditional medicine have been operating smoking cessation clinics since the early 1990s, especially in the acupuncture divisions of university hospitals. Reports on the effects of ear treatment have been released since 1992. One paper coming out that year reported a complete cessation rate of 40.5 percent, with 82 percent of patients reducing their smoking 75 percent or more after four or more treatments.

Moxibustion

A lesser-known treatment is moxibustion, which applies mugwort to areas of the body and then burns the herb to provide remedial benefits through heat stimulation and infusion of mugwort ingredients. Moxibustion is thought to have originated in primitive times, when clumps of twigs or grass were likely used. Over time, mugwort emerged as the primary ingredient according to China's oldest medical text, *Huangdi Neijing*, written in the Han Dynasty (3rd century B.C.–A.D. 3rd century), which includes a reference to "treatment with needles and mugwort."

Mugwort is harvested annually from March to May. Fresh and thick-stemmed mugwort plants are gathered, dried in the sun, and ground into a powder with a mortar and pestle. This coarse powder is passed through a sieve to remove any stems or foreign objects several times until only a refined mugwort powder remains. The powder, known as moxa, is tamped into a mold to produce small cone-shaped forms.

Moxibustion treatment utilizes the heat from the burning of moxa cones and infusion of mugwort's ingredients, which affect the

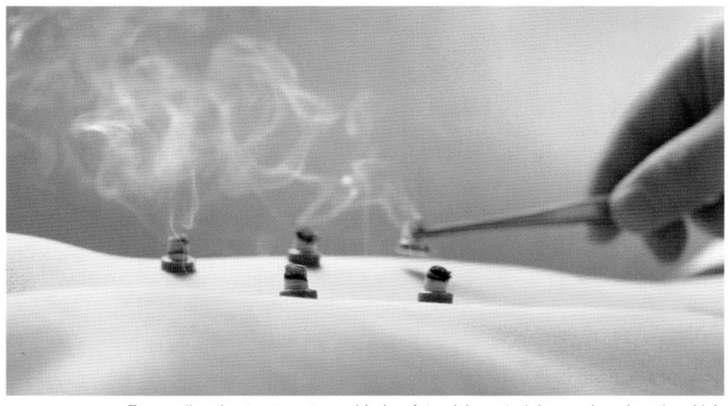

For moxibustion treatment, smoldering Artemisia materials are placed on the skin's surface to provide heat therapy and energy stimulation.

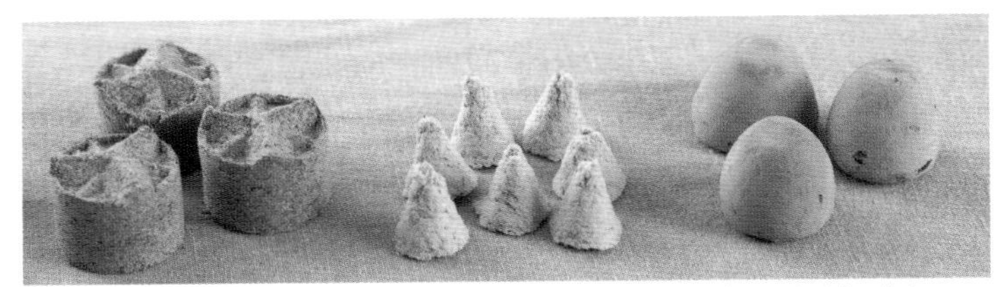
A wide variety of moxibustion therapy materials are available at pharmacies and retail outlets.

entire body. This process can help improve blood circulation and metabolism, eliminate negative energy, and boost positive energy in addition to relieving fever and providing warmth. Moxibustion treatment includes direct and indirect applications. For direct application, the bottom of a moxa cone is placed onto the skin surface and burned, whereas for indirect treatment, the subject area is first covered with another material such as a paste of soybean, ginger, garlic, yellow earth, or salt. Above all, careful attention is necessary to prevent burning the skin of a patient, who might fall asleep or experience loss of sensation. Even with indirect treatment, the heat must be regulated to prevent blistering. Direct moxibustion is also not applied to the face or abdomen of a pregnant woman or for a patient with a cold.

Herbal Medicine

Hanyak, or Korean herbal medicine, is often thought to be associated with folk remedies. But Korean traditional medicine is entirely different. Whereas a folk remedy might identify a particular herb used to treat an ailment, Korean traditional medicine represents a pharmacological system of treatment based on long-term clinical research.

The ingredients included in a prescription of herbal medicine are determined by the desired effect. Medicinal ingredients used in

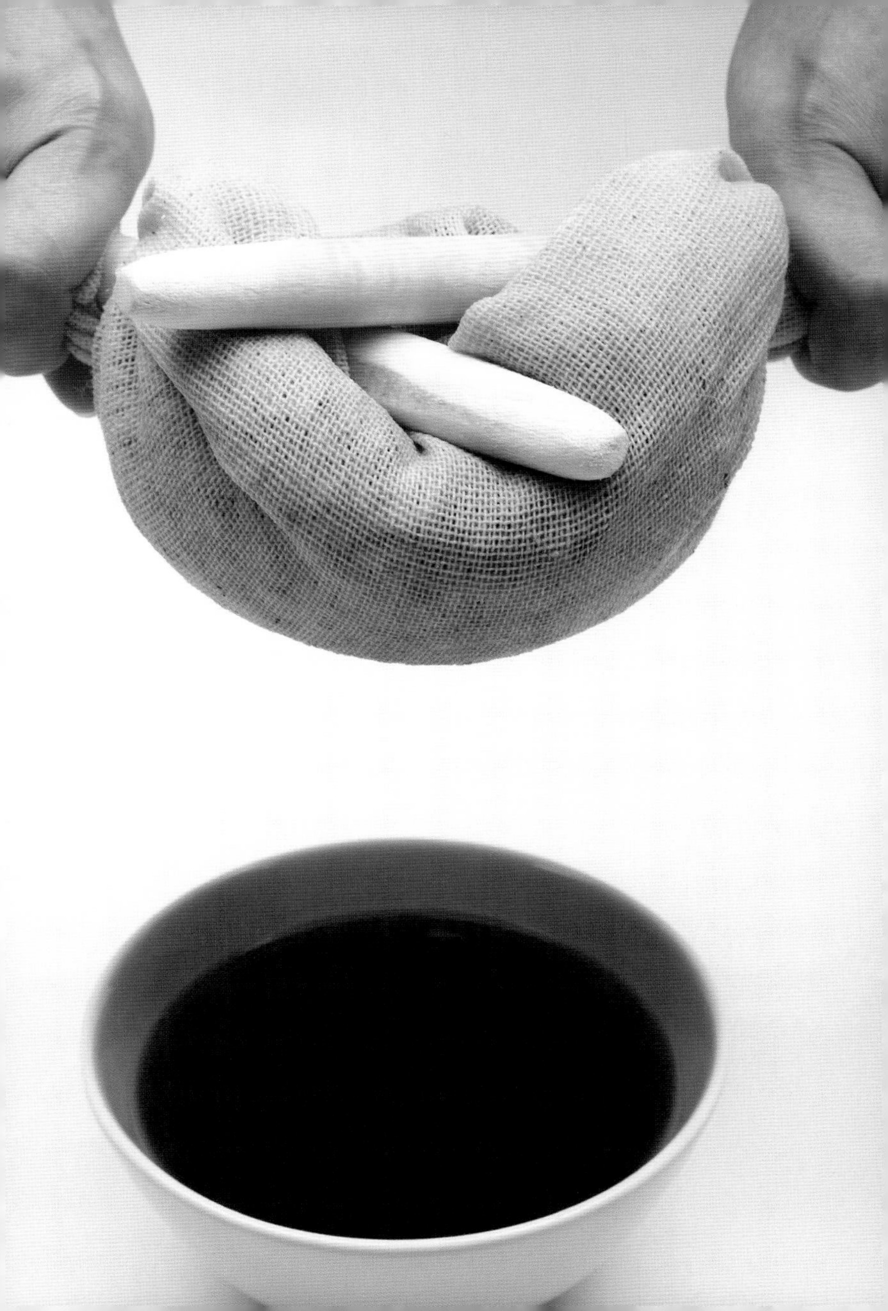

Herbal Ingredients

Ingredients from natural plants, animals, and minerals are used to prevent and treat illness in accordance with the principles of Korean traditional medicine. One important type, *yakcho*, consists of plants harvested and used in their natural state. These *yakcho* herbs are typically dried in the sun or shade, painstakingly selected, and cut or ground into a powder for medicinal use. The entire plant may be used for medicine, or the roots, stem, bark, leaves, fruits, and seeds may be applied. The list of herbs used in Korean traditional medicine is very long, but the following are among the most common:

- **Licorice (*gamcho*):** This is a mild herb, neither warm nor cold, with a sweet flavor that grows in the wild in China, Mongolia, and Uzbekistan, and is widely cultivated in Korea. Licorice is highly effective in cleansing toxins and supplementing weaknesses in spleen and stomach functions; when roasted with honey, it provides an excellent supplement for people experiencing physical weakness. When used raw, it can be applied externally as an effective treatment for boils.

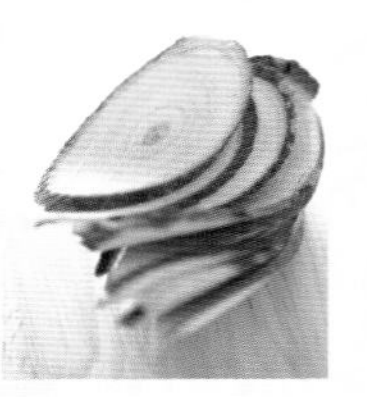

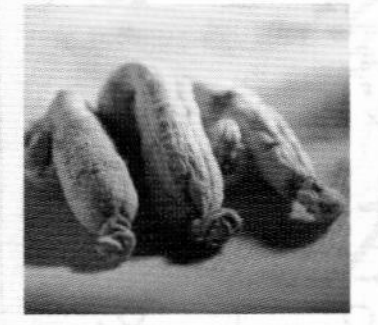

- **Ginseng (*insam*):** The effects of Korean ginseng are renowned the world over, with a rich body of research on its components. Ginseng helps maintain homeostasis in the body, strengthens bodily functions, stimulates the nervous system, promotes the functions of the pituitary gland and adrenocortical hormones, bolsters immunity, boosts sexual function, strengthens the heart, encourages digestion, accelerates metabolism, builds appetite, stabilizes nerves, and alleviates asthma. Ginseng is often used in the event of sudden shock, cold hands and/or feet, particular susceptibity to the cold, lack of energy, or weak digestive organs. It has also proven outstandingly effective in strengthening immune and cardiac functions, forming blood, fighting cancer, and lowering blood sugar.

- **Mugwort (*ssuk/aeyeop*):** Mugwort is a warm herb with a bitter, spicy flavor that is often effective in stopping hemorrhage and treating pain. In the former, the herb is used to treat various types of bleeding including cold weather hematemesis (vomiting of blood), hemoptysis (coughing up blood from the lungs), and nasal

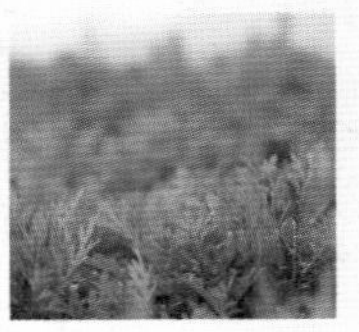

bleeding. It is also applied to pain experienced during a period and menstrual irregularities resulting from coldness in the lower abdomen, and can calm the movements of a fetus in the womb or relieve abdominal pains. Externally, mugwort is useful against eczema and itching, often in the form of moxa.

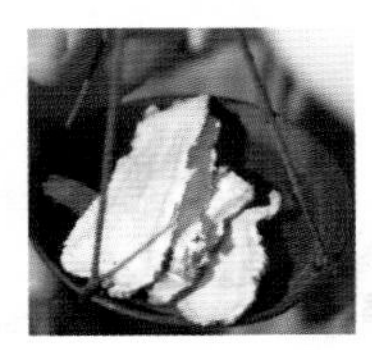

• **Angelica root (*danggwi*):** The effects of angelica root depend on the part of the root used. The ascending top portion can be used to stop bleeding. The middle portion also stops bleeding, while the descending bottom portion dissolves clots in the blood. More generally, the root harmonizes with the blood and promotes circulation. Angelica root is one of most commonly prescribed herbs for women's ailments, especially menstrual irregularities and period pains, but also used for ailments related to poor circulation and lack of blood including headaches, stomach pain, dizziness, constipation, weakened digestion, bruising, sprains, various types of bleeding, and swelling.

• **Kudzu root (*galgeun*):** Kudzu root promotes sweating, which helps to relax muscles. It is used to relieve colds, a sickness associated with chills and fever that prevent sweating and cause stiffness in the neck and back of the head, and dysentery, which can sometimes arise as a complication of the cold. Because the root helps produce essence and stops thirst, it is also used to treat diabetes and sometimes applied to stop diarrhea and dysentery. The flowers of the kudzu plant can also be used as herbs. Called *galhwa*, the flowers help relieve alcohol poisoning and are used to treat liver ailments and stomach damage from drinking.

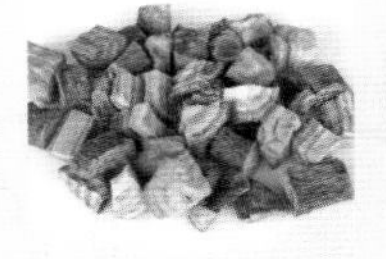

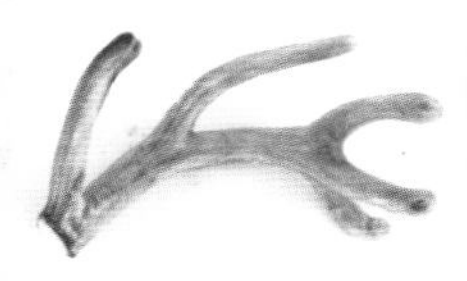

• **Deer antler (*nogyong*):** Every spring, the deer sheds its antlers and grows a soft new set in their place. These are removed and used as an ingredient called *nogyong*. Another product from antlers is *nokgak*, which are the hard, bony hairs that fall out of the antlers when they are left to grow. Antler products are used to promote growth and blood creation, strengthen the heart, and bolster immunity.

Korean traditional medicine each have a variety of effects. For example, ginseng is effective in providing warmth, reinforcing the body's energy flow, relieving fatigue, bolstering the immune system, soothing anxiety, aiding digestion and quenching thirst. The ingredients of herbal medicine are commonly categorized by four characteristics—hot, warm, cool, and cold—and five tastes—sour, bitter, sweet, spicy, and salty.

According to Western science, the active ingredients of medicine are what matters most. On the other hand, in Korean traditional medicine, the efficacy of a prescribed medicine is maximized by properly combining a number of separate ingredients. In situations when Korean traditional medicine alone is not effective, Western medicine can also be applied to produce a more powerful treatment. This has long been a common practice in Korea, but the combination of Eastern and Western treatment has gained increasing popularity in Japan as well.

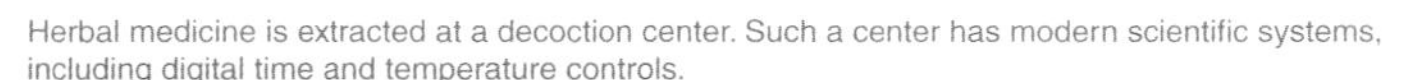

Herbal medicine is extracted at a decoction center. Such a center has modern scientific systems, including digital time and temperature controls.

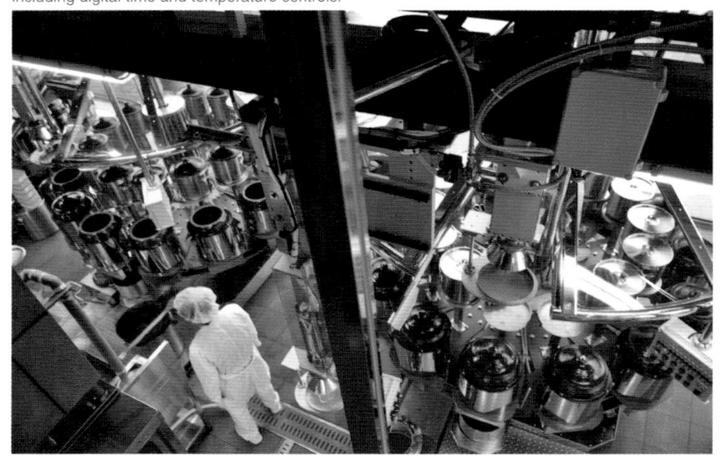

Because of the natural ingredients of herbal medicine, *hanyak* is dispensed in a wide variety of forms. For example, herbal decoctions are produced by boiling herbal ingredients in water and retaining the liquid primarily for use against serious diseases. Medicine in powdered form is usually made by grinding up dry ingredients, which can be combined with a filler material such as flour and honey, and shaped into round pills for more convenient handling and portability. Distilled medicine, which is often prescribed to treat illness in young children, is obtained by collecting a specified amount of steam from boiling medicinal ingredients. In addition, extract forms are the result of boiling ingredients, allowing the moisture to evaporate, and freeze-drying the residue. For skin disorders and boils, an adhesive patch coated with powdered ingredients is applied to the problem areas.

Today, Korean herbal medicine is manufactured under commercial processes similar to that of Western-style medicine to facilitate easier use by consumers. This includes herbal-based capsules, liquid forms, patches for joint and muscle pain, ointments, creams, and sprays.

Other Treatments

Cupping

Cupping is the application of small bowl-shaped cups to the surface of the body as a way of removing harmful elements. The process uses negative pressure generated by removing the air inside.

Exactly when cupping began remains unknown, but it has been part of both Eastern and Western medicine since time immemorial. Older methods used animal horns and bamboo, but the latest manner generates negative pressure either manually or electrically. Cupping is used to treat not only external ailments like bruising,

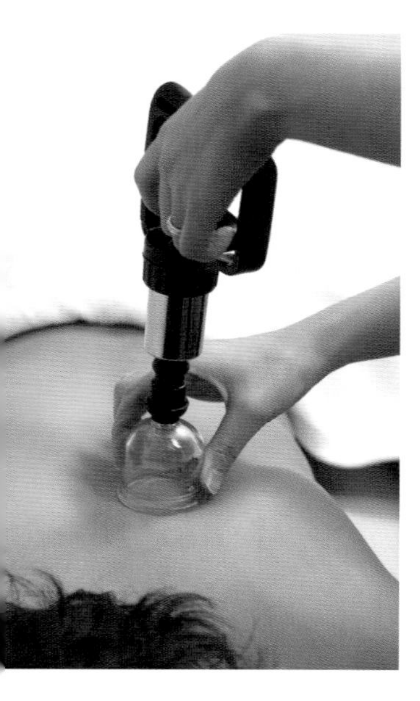

but also a wide range of chronic internal conditions.

Cupping has two main types: wet and dry. Wet cupping is used to remove blood and other bodily fluids, while dry cupping simply applies negative pressure to a body part without releasing any fluids. The principle behind dry cupping is that because the skin's surface allows the passage of gases but not blood, it should be possible to cleanse fluids through the gas exchange that occurs due to the pressure differential when negative pressure is applied.

The primary effects of cupping are seen in metabolism and blood purification, thanks to the gas exchange. A second effect is the promotion of blood circulation and formation, while a third is the distribution of nutrients to the cells and excretion of waste matter and toxins. Cupping is also known to be effective in adjusting the acid/base balance in bodily fluids and boosting immune function.

Chuna

The technique known as chuna falls into the category of external treatment, with the physician treating the patient through use of the hands. The effects result from adjustments to the body's physiological and pathological conditions by manipulation of certain parts of the body—acupoints, tender spots on the fascia, the spine and joints—with the hands, other parts of the body, or equipment.

This has two effects. First, the physician adjusts the body's

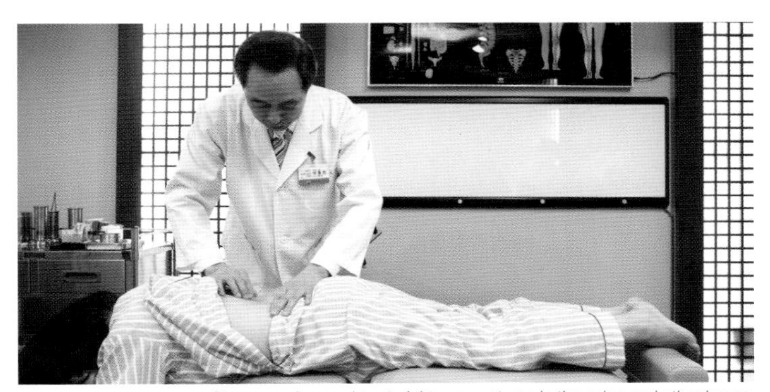

Chuna can be used to straighten curvatures in the spine and other bones.

balance by straightening anatomical positions. Second, the dynamic waves from the use of the hands are converted into a kind of energy that permeates deep into the body and the relevant tissues and organs. Benefits of chuna include the avoidance of toxins and side effects associated with medications, helping the patient feel immediate comfort in the treatment process, and its effectiveness in treating a wide range of ailments.

Aromatherapy

Aromatherapy is a form of natural medicine that uses fragrant oils extracted from leaves, roots, fruits, and petals. The scents produce effects when introduced through inhalation, bathing, or massage. The use of aromatherapy techniques based on the principles of Korean traditional medicine first grew prevalent thanks to the efforts of the Korean Oriental Medicine Naturopathy Institute (founded in 1996). Today, the subject is widely researched by think tanks around the world, including many in the West, with a number of reports showing positive treatment effects.

Aromatherapy is based on the principle that small airborne

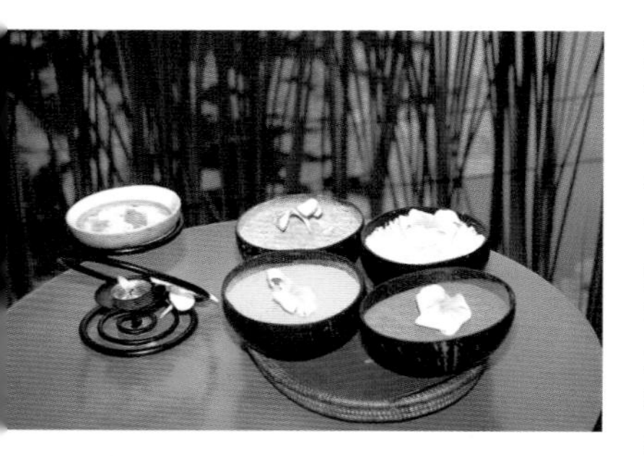

particles inhaled through the nose will have different effects on the brain depending on shape. The ones that go to the limbic system will be analyzed by the brain and produce neurochemical substances to promote calm, relax tension, provide stimulation, and improve mood. All of this contributes to maintaining overall health. The method has been especially effective in skin care and the treatment of insomnia, depression, skin conditions, period pains, and rhinitis.

Taping

Taping is another method that treats disease without the use of medication. The physician applies tape to particular muscles or meridians and acupoints. The stimulation helps the flow of energy and blood to proceed more smoothly and corrects the body's balance by treating the tension and release of muscles, tendons, and ligaments. Taping has proven effective in treating a range of musculoskeletal conditions, including chronic degenerative disc disease in the neck and lower back, degenerative arthritis, frozen shoulder, ankylosing spondylitis, vertebral pressure fractures (especially in the elderly), and spinal stenosis. It has also been used to treat constipation, digestive disorders, headaches, and insomnia and strengthen the muscles and prevent muscle problems.

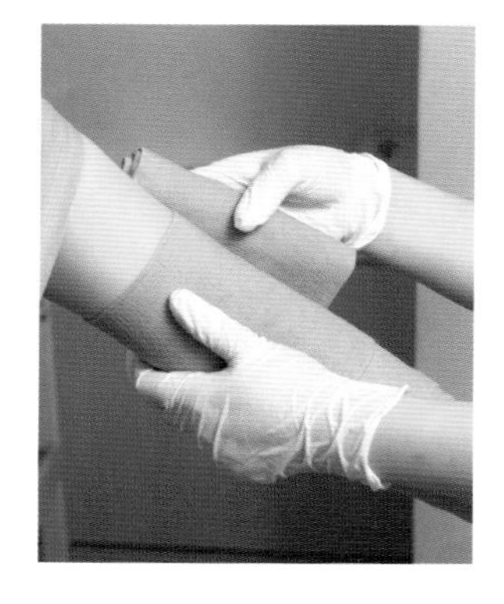

Medicine Markets: Yangnyeongsi

Yangnyeongsi began in the second year of the reign of King Hyojong (r. 1650–1659), the 17th monarch of the Joseon Dynasty. For nearly 300 years until 1943 (toward the end of Japanese colonial rule of Korea), the markets specialized in Korean medicinal ingredients. Before they were created, people who wanted such ingredients usually had to venture into the mountains to find them. They often spent half the year finding the plants and the other half selling them. Patients with particularly acute conditions ended up dying because no medicine was available. To tackle this problem, *Yangnyeongsi* was founded as part of a deliberate effort by the state. The idea was to create venues where people could find the medicine they needed more easily and quickly. Markets were set up in central locations, allowing for ease of harvesting and traffic between regions. The first markets were built in Daegu, Wonju, and Jeonju because they were the respective centers of the provinces of Gyeongsang, Gangwon, and Jeolla, where most of the medicines were produced. Typically, the markets were held twice a year, in the spring and fall.

- **Daegu Yangnyeongsi:** The Daegu market was the busiest of all. Set up in the days of King Hyojong, the seasonal market was staged regularly in the spring and fall. The reason it was only open those two seasons is they were the times

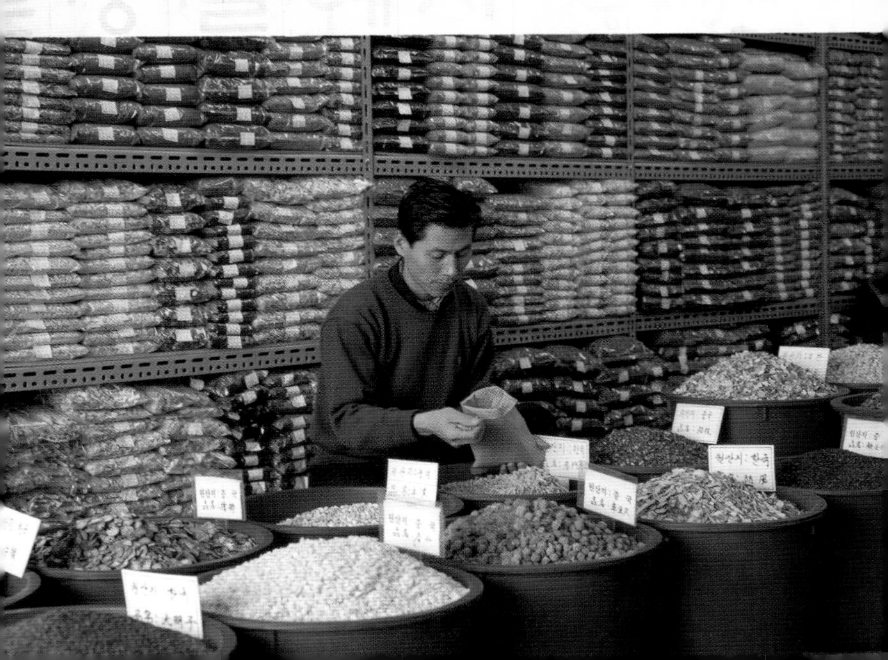

of year when the medicines were harvested. For centuries, the market enjoyed an excellent reputation in Korea and abroad, but began to decline in importance after the Japanese occupied Korea. After the country was liberated from colonial rule, *hanyak* (herbal medicine) sellers decided to revive the *yangnyeongsi* tradition as an example of the nation's cultural heritage. Thanks to these efforts, the markets were opened once again, but the outbreak of the Korean War resulted in most of them shutting down. It was not until 1978 that another revival came, courtesy of the Daegu Herbal Medicine Association. The result of this was the founding of the Yangnyeongsi Preservation Committee. Today, an herbal medicine festival is held every spring and an *yangnyeongsi* culture festival in October, Korea's national culture month.

- **Jeonju Yangnyeongsi:** Second only to the Daegu market in scale, the Jeonju Yangnyeongsi was organized at a major transit point for valuable medicines from the surrounding area, especially Mt. Jirisan and Jeju Island. It was established around November 1932 and lasted for three months, from October 1 until late December by the lunar calendar. The ingredients traded there were produced in regions with the best natural conditions including Mt. Jirisan, Mt. Deogyusan, Mt. Naejangsan, and the Byeonsanbando Peninsula. In addition to having the best quality of medicines, the market also boasted a number of rare ones found nowhere else.

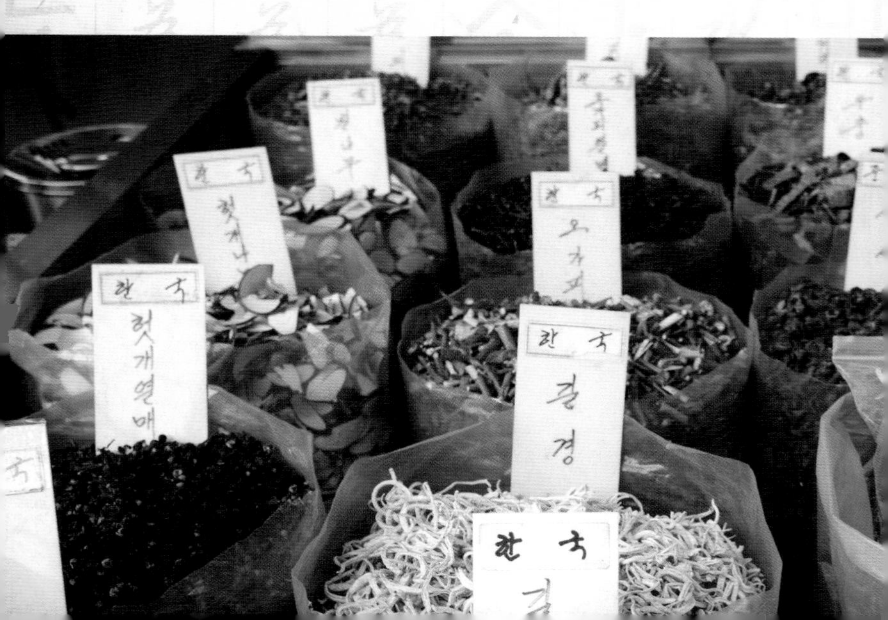

- **Seoul (Gyeongdong) Yangnyeongsi:** The area known today as Seoul Yangnyeongsi, located in central Seoul's Dongdaemun district, was once home to Bojewon, a center designated by the city as its 23rd historic site. During the Joseon era, Bojewon was a relief organization offering free lodging and treatment to the sick who had nowhere else to go. This spirit had a major influence on Joseon-era Korea in general, and the center carried on the tradition with developments in folk medicine.

  Today, the market is a national center for Korean traditional medicine. It was organized more or less spontaneously in the 1960s, helped in no small part by the prime location it occupied. On June 1, 1995, a section of the market was designated by the city as Gyeongdong Yangnyeongsi, a center specializing in *hanyak*. As of 2000, it was a major *hanyak* hub, accounting for around 70 percent of all transactions nationwide and home to around 330 clinics and 930 *hanyak* businesses.

  In the late 1960s, the market was transformed into that for specialized products. By the end of the next decade, it had become firmly established as a national center specializing in Korean medicinal ingredients. In 1983, it began dealing in ginseng and honey. Today, an estimated three-fourths of all ginseng and honey consumed in Seoul and about two-thirds of all Korean herbal medicine in the country go through this market.

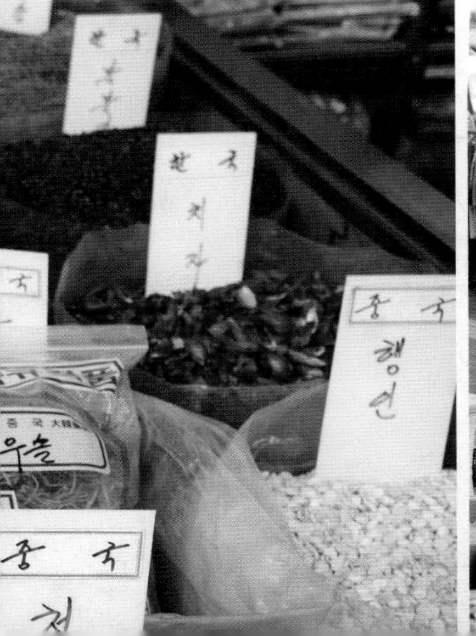

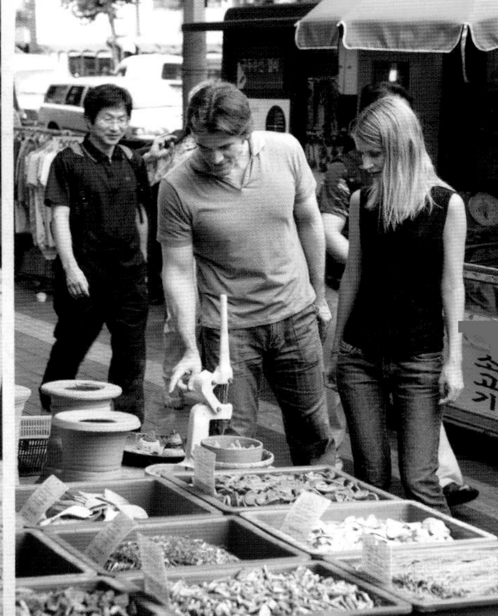

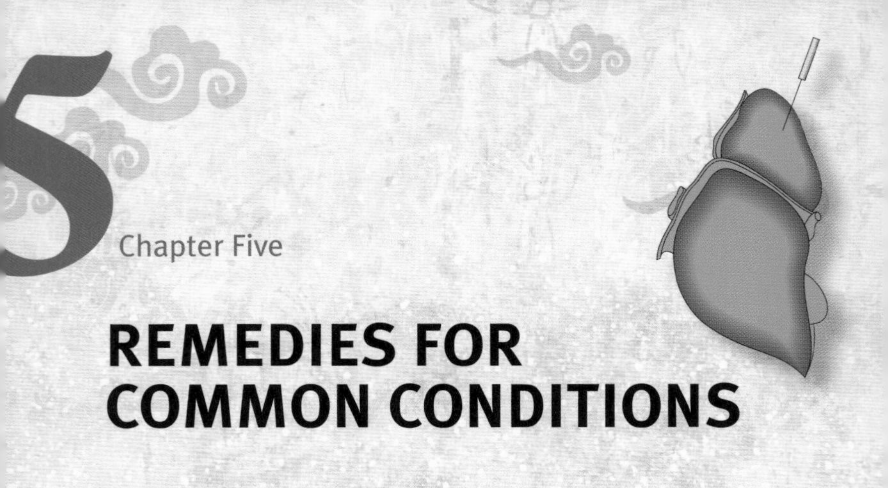

Chapter Five

REMEDIES FOR COMMON CONDITIONS

COLD

The cold is caused by viruses of a great many types, including rhinoviruses and adenoviruses to name just two. Each of them is associated with different symptoms: sneezing, stuffy or runny nose, sore throat, coughing, fever, headaches, and muscle pain. So far, no medicine has been developed that can kill cold viruses. The primary approach in Western medicine is to treat the symptoms, with antibiotics prescribed in the case of secondary inflammation. But the only thing that can neutralize cold viruses is the body's own immune system. This means that the best approach for people who suffer from frequent or persistent colds is to strengthen that system. In Korean traditional medicine, treatment is focused on both eliminating bad energy that invades from outside and bolstering the body's immune functions.

The earliest symptoms of a cold-chills, runny or stuffy nose, sneezing—are signs that bad energy has not penetrated deep into the body but is making its way inside. Often, all that is needed to relieve them is giving the body strength enough to fight them off, either by reducing fatigue or increasing nutrients. One good method to do this is to warm the body with ginger or citron tea. A green onion root concoction is another effective option.

Once the cold has progressed and symptoms appear like coughing, heavy phlegm, fever, and pain in the head and body, this means bad energy has penetrated deeply and rest is no longer sufficient to fight it. In this case, the symptoms can be relieved by supplementing the patient's own right energy so that it can expel bad energy from the body. After bad energy is gone, the patient is often given medicine to boost immune function to prevent against frequent colds. Even if he or she catches cold again, it will be minor and short-lived if bad energy is expelled from the body.

Jujube tea is considered an excellent remedy for colds and insomnia.

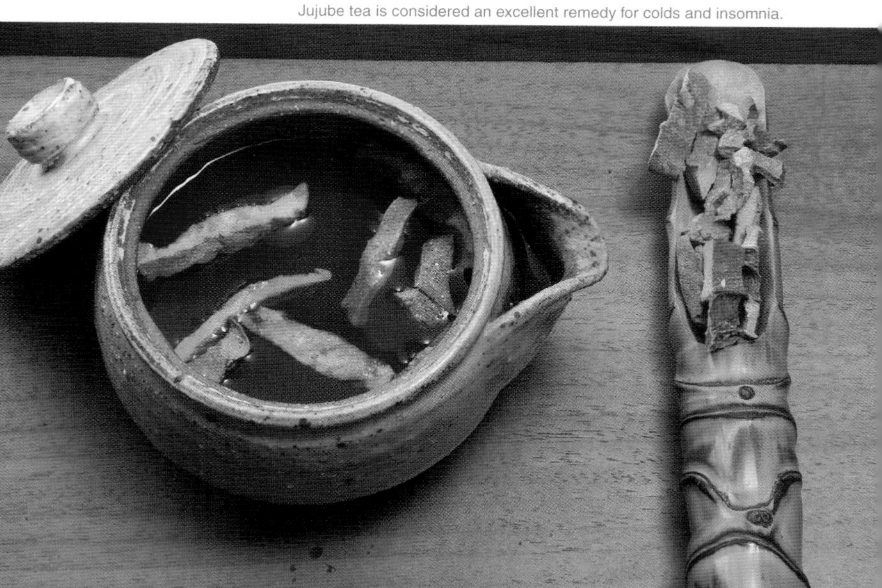

Menopausal Syndrome

When the body's five viscera and six bowels are working normally, the upper part of the body (head and chest) is cool, while the bottom half is warm. As people grow older and experience physical weakening and stress, internal organs have more difficulty functioning and begin to generate heat. Heat rises, so the upper body begins to grow warmer and the bottom half grows cooler under a phenor[illegible]lled *sangyeolhahan* in Korean traditional medicine. Resul[illegible] include symptoms like blushing, headache, dizziness, chest [illegible]ion, sleeping difficulty, anxiety, depression, diminished sexual function, and frequent urination. Since these are especially common in women who are beginning menopause, this class of conditions has been called "menopausal syndrome."

In Western medicine, these symptoms are seen as resulting from lack of female hormones, but Korean traditional medicine blames an excess of pent-up anger in the heart and liver. In other words, heart and liver energy becomes uncomfortable and stagnant, which causes heat in the upper body, and the aforementioned symptoms are the result. Bringing down the temperature means releasing pent-up energy in the heart and liver with supplementation of right energy in the kidneys used to boost energy in the lower body.

Headaches

Headaches are one of the most common ailments around. They affect everyone, young and old. Some are more severe than others, and many suffer from chronic headaches with no discernible cause. Korean traditional medicine has proven effective in treating chronic headaches without the use of surgery or emergency medical intervention. Even in cases where testing fails to uncover a cause, practitioners of Korean traditional medicine believe there is both a cause and appropriate treatment for every symptom and body type.

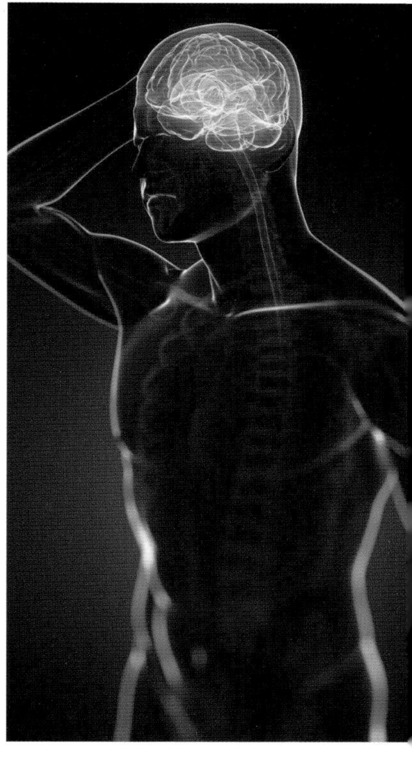

In Korean traditional medicine, headaches are seen not as a disease of the head itself, but a cumulative failure to achieve harmony in general bodily functions. The same types of headache might have different symptoms and causes.

The different causes can be seen in the types of pain experienced by the patient. Stabbing headaches are caused by bruising or lack of blood circulation, as well as headaches caused by buildup of unnecessary moisture and non-circulating fluids characterized by grogginess and a heavy feeling like something is on top of the patient's head.

Headaches are also distinguished by the place where pain is felt. A phlegm-retention headache is characterized by excruciating pain radiating from the eyes to the crown of the head, dizziness, general heaviness in the body, coldness in the extremities, and queasiness. A blood weakness headache, in contrast, is characterized by pain from the outside of the eyebrows and is accompanied by paleness, rapid heartbeat, and increased startle reflex.

Another way to distinguish causes is the time when pain is experienced. Headaches that occur in the morning are associated with weakness of blood and energy, while serious headaches in the afternoon and evening are associated with weakness of *yin* energy.

Different types require different treatments. The best method in the early stages is often acupuncture alone, while chronic headaches require a combination of acupuncture and herbal medicine.

Melancholy and Rage

Korean traditional medicine has identified a number of conditions associated with severe stress, including melancholy, rage, and a combination of the two. Melancholy is quite similar to the modern concept of depression; it refers to a condition resulting from psychological causes in which energy remains clustered inside the body. Rage originates in the heart and is associated with emotions of anger. A person who leaves these emotions bottled inside will eventually explode in anger. The concept might be seen as analogous to anxiety disorders or neurosis in modern psychological terms.

Following the principle that body and mind form an inseparable whole, Korean traditional medicine emphasizes the relationship between the five viscera and psychological aspects contained within each organ. Treatment focuses on improving mental function through adjustment and strengthening of the viscera. Indeed, psychological functions frequently manifest themselves in the form of warmth in the upper body, digestive disorders, insomnia, headache, dizziness, and a constricted feeling in the chest. The physician tries to improve mental as well as physical condition, treating the symptoms in the body while also working to fix the balance in the viscera.

For a patient suffering from melancholy, treatment typically uses herbs such as bupleurum, nut grass, citrus peel extract, elecampane,

Natural herbs used to prepare herbal medicine

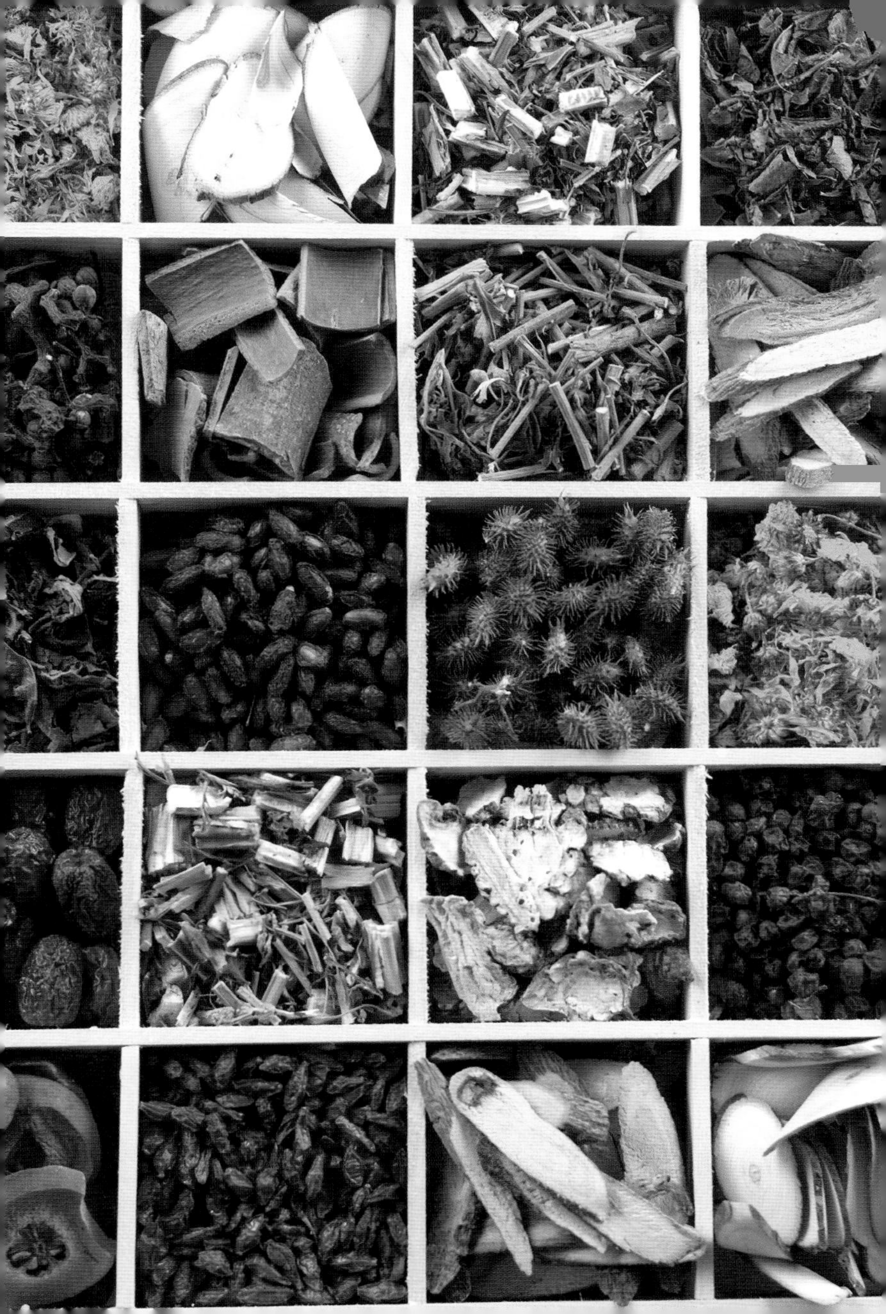

or lindera root to promote energy flow. The aim is to dislodge the energy that is failing to circulate. Rage, which is viewed as resulting from an upward surge of anger in the heart, is treated with acupuncture to bring the heat back down. The heat is also treated with medications, including herbs like sacred lotus, gardenia seeds, snake's beard, or bamboo shavings.

CHRONIC FATIGUE

The term *dubulcheong*—literally, "unclear head"—is used in Korean traditional medicine to describe a kind of fatigue characterized by a continued feeling of daze that does not improve with rest. The condition is seen as resulting from three possible causes.

The first cause is the inability of clear energy to go where it needs to. Korean traditional medicine identifies clear and thick energies in the spleen and stomach (i.e., the viscera and bowels in charge of digestion) when eating food. Clear energy rises to the head to assist mental function, while thick energy descends in the form of urine and feces. When spleen and stomach functions are diminished and the two types of energy cannot be distinguished, the result can be a sense of dullness and fatigue.

The second cause is unnecessary waste products such as stagnated blood or congested fluids in the body preventing clear energy from rising to the upper body. In this case, prescriptions include herbs to eliminate stagnated blood (angelica root, peachseed, safflower, and chuan xiong) or congested fluids (crow dipper, citrus peel, and bai zhu).

The final cause is a general reduction of bodily strength. When a patient experiences both dullness in the head and fatigue that does not improve with sleep, the condition requires a full-body diagnosis.

Conditions Related to Pregnancy, Childbirth, and Postpartum Treatmen

In Korean traditional medicine, sterility, or the inability to conceive a child, is seen as resulting from a number of factors such as weakness of the kidneys, congestion of the liver, damp phlegm, and blood deficiency. The first two are similar to the kind of hormonal disorders described in Western medicine, while damp phlegm in the body is associated with sterility resulting from pathogens entering the body. When the cause is blood deficiency, the condition results from weakness in the body. Suitable treatments prescribed for each of these causes include acupuncture, herbal medications, and moxibustion.

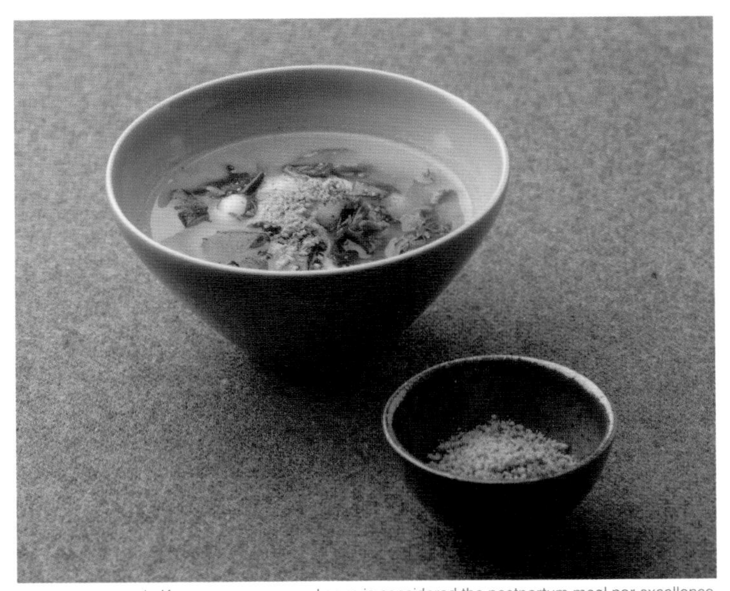

In Korea, green seaweed soup is considered the postpartum meal par excellence.

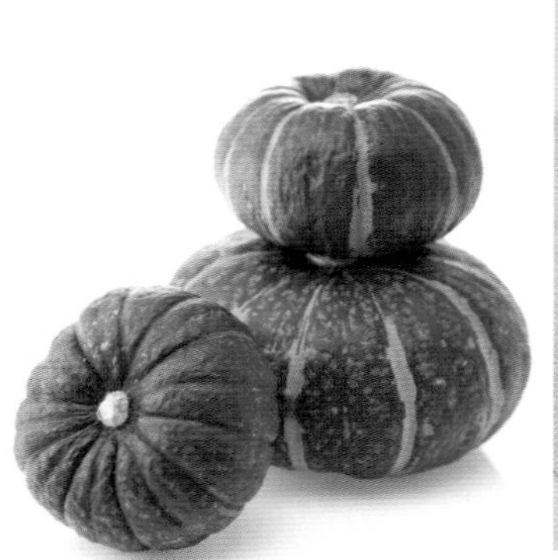

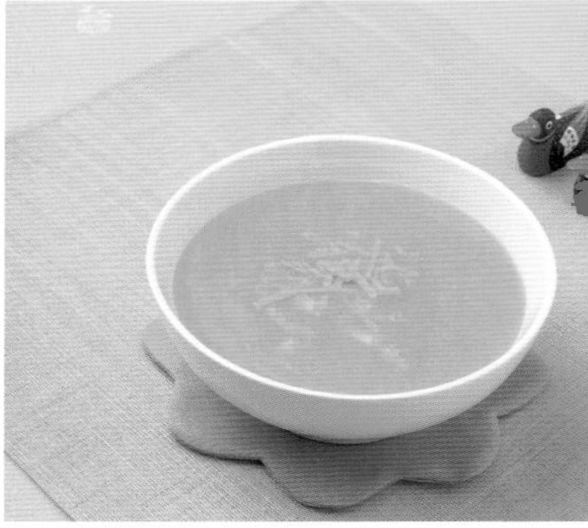

Pumpkin porridge has excellent diuretic effects and is good for treating postpartum edema.

The most common treatment when childbirth is expected to be difficult is *dalsaengsan*, which is often called "medicine for a safe delivery." *Dalsaengsan*, which was mentioned as far back as the time of *Donguibogam*, is prescribed in the later stages of pregnancy to reduce amniotic fluid for easier delivery. By slightly reducing the size of the fluid-swollen baby, it allows for easier passage through the uterus. A report presented in an academic conference said the average time of childbirth was reduced 40 percent or more with the use of *dalsaengsan*. Another medication called *bulsusan* is also prescribed when childbirth is imminent. This increases the contractile force of the uterus and reduces the time of labor pain, while relaxing muscles to help the uterus open more easily. Both medicines are used for easier and safer childbirth but cannot be used indiscriminately. The dose should be adjusted according to the mother's condition and body type and the symptoms she exhibits.

In the postpartum recovery period, it is important to make up for energy and blood damage from the childbirth process and help the mother return to her pre-pregnancy condition as soon as possible. While the situations of patients vary, most women experience lochia, or the release of secretions from wounds to the endometrium from the shedding of placenta and ovaries. Treatment involves prescriptions to restore energy and blood and push lochia out more easily. Medications also help to relieve swelling and promote milk flow.

In addition to the medications, the mother should eat a wide range of foods. Green seaweed is considered the best food for women recovering from childbirth; it assists in uterine contractions, clears the blood, and helps restore joint functions. Pumpkin is another excellent choice; it helps metabolize fluids while its diuretic effects relieve edema. It also strengthens overall energy by promoting digestion.

Hair Loss

A healthy head of hair requires healthy organs and a good supply of oxygen and nutrients to the scalp. The hair's owner also needs to eliminate waste matter. For this reason, effective hair loss treatment requires smooth circulation and a sufficient supply of energy and blood. In Korean traditional medicine, hair loss is associated with the functions of a number of internal organs, with different treatments prescribed accordingly.

The spleen is a digestive organ that processes the fluids and nutrients the body absorbs, converts them into purer forms, and delivers these substances to other organs that need them. When a diet is too strict or nutrition poor, the hair tends to weaken and grows thin and brittle, and these characteristics are associated with the spleen. To relieve these symptoms, a healthy, functioning spleen is important.

In Korean traditional medicine, the lungs are not only associated with respiratory organs like bronchial tubes and nose, they are also seen as affecting the skin and hair. So for healthy and shiny hair, both nutrients and fresh air, which means healthy lungs, are needed. This is why people undergoing hair loss treatment also tend to see improvement in rhinitis and asthma and acquire healthier skin.

The kidneys keep hair healthy and dark through the blood. But as people age and their kidney function diminishes, they often lose their hair or see it turn prematurely gray. When hair loss and aging occur around menopause, the treatment typically seeks to boost kidney function.

Steam Bidet Therapy

Steam bidet therapy involves boiling herbs in water and applying the steam to reproductive organs to boost warmth in that region of the body. The herbs help to kill pathogens, quench heat, and promote circulation of the blood and energy, and the bidet also helps to shrink the lower abdomen by eliminating part of the waste matter and unnecessary fat that has built up there.

This approach is especially effective for people with obesity in their lower body. The problem is a vicious cycle in which abdominal fat causes coldness in the lower abdomen, which then leads to more abdominal fat as a way of protecting the cold area. Both steam bidets and moxibustion help fight abdominal obesity by warming the abdomen. The bidets are also good for women suffering from cold-related conditions, with applications including leucorrhea, genital itching, coldness in the lower abdomen, bladder infection, and sterility. They can also be used for hemorrhoids and anal prolapse since they unblock blood around the anus and strengthen weakened muscles.

Steam bidets are considered an integral part of Korean traditional medicine. Sources like *Donguibogam* prescribe steam treatment for ailments of a woman's lower abdomen, which are seen as resulting from cold energy. A

As an organ, the liver is responsible for storing blood, eliminating toxins, and ensuring a supply of clean blood to the body. If the health of hair is closely tied to a supply of clean blood, then the key to keeping it healthy is maintaining a healthy liver.

In women, the uterus is seen as governing the blood. In many cases, hair loss in women is associated with uterine health. Women also tend to suffer from irregular menstruation, period pains, leucorrhea, and ovulation discomfort, along with coldness in the extremities and redness in the face. Any treatment must start by making the uterus healthy and functioning.

---

patient requires continuous treatment, and even healthy people can benefit from the disease prevention effects of regular bidet therapy.

The herbs used in bidets include mugwort, which is good for warming the body; dandelion, which is effective at killing germs and promoting circulation to reduce abdominal fat; and Chinese motherwort, which is used to treat pain during a period and menstrual irregularities.

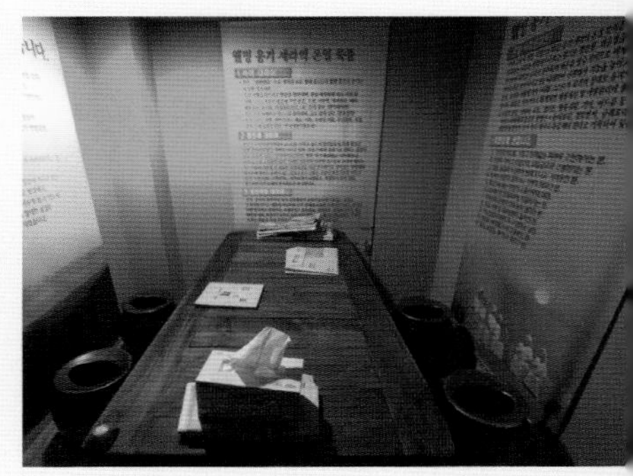
The steam bidet room is designed for ease of treatment.

The process, however, does require caution. Cleanliness is essential since the process involves applying steam directly to the reproductive area. People undergoing the treatment must keep their area clean and dry both before and after the treatment. One treatment typically takes 15–20 minutes, and the most optimal course is to have three treatments per week.

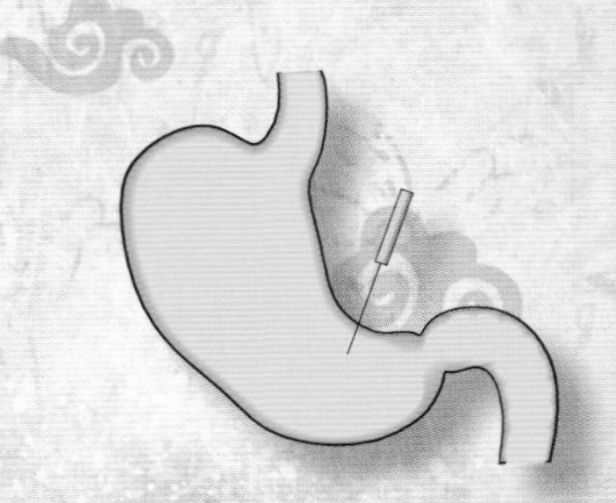

Chapter Six

KOREAN MEDICINE TODAY AND TOMORROW

Korean traditional medicine is often described as "experiential medicine," but is a science founded in a complete theory based on the principles of birth and nature. The reason such medicine is more misunderstood than its Western counterpart is because the mechanisms of the former's treatment have not been demonstrated using modern analytical technology. Decades after Western medical techniques and other examples of Western civilization were introduced in the Korean Enlightenment period, the field was dismissed as "folk wisdom." But it has made a comeback in recent years, thanks to the efforts of doctors of Korean traditional medicine and growing Western interest in a holistic medical approach and natural remedies. The revival has also been bolstered by the popularization of herbal medicine, establishment of colleges of Korean traditional medicine, development of specialized treatments in specialized areas, diagnostic techniques using state-of-the-art medical equipment, changes in the types of drugs (distillations, powders, capsules and concentrate), development of forms for external application, and research tied to the emerging field of bioengineering.

New Trends

Korean traditional medicine over the centuries has held that the doctor must examine the patient's body as a whole when treating even a single, localized ailment. Because of this, doctors usually did not specialize in specific areas of treatment.

Recently, however, specialization has become more of a trend among Korean traditional medicine providers mainly due to the growing market for traditional medicine and heavier competition. Since 2002, such practitioners have chosen one of eight areas of

A foreign athlete in Korea for a taekwondo competition is examined with state-of-the-art equipment at a Korean traditional medicine clinic.

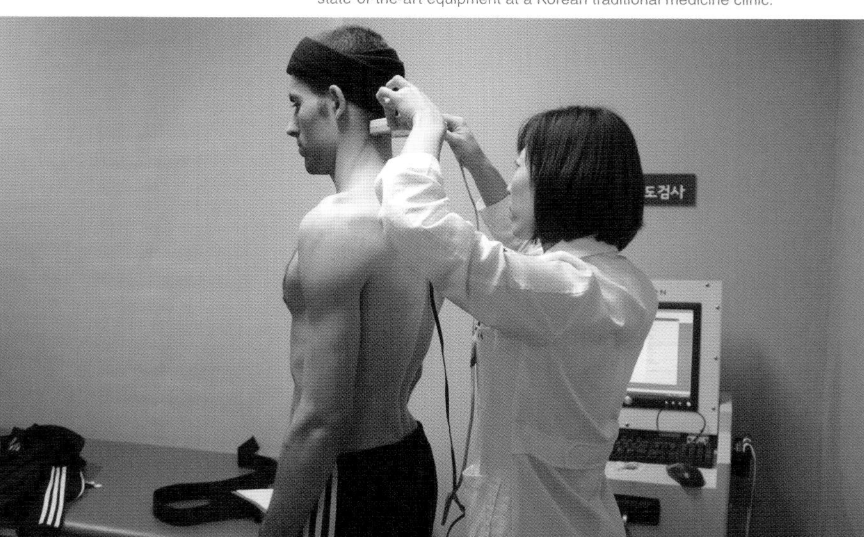

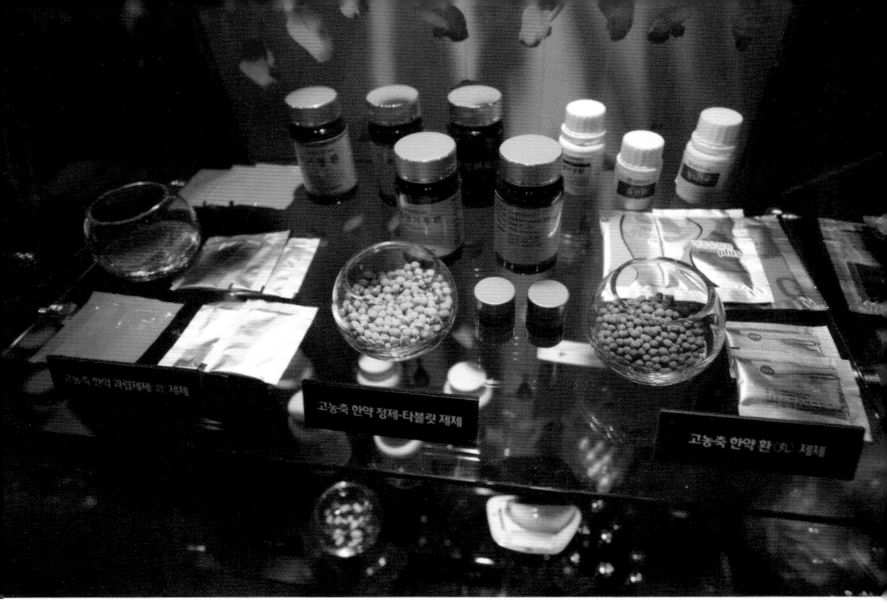

Different kinds of herbal medicine have been developed in recent years.

specialization: internal medicine, acupuncture, rehabilitation medicine, obstetrics/gynecology, pediatrics, the four constitutions, otorhinolaryngology, and neurology. Specialized institutions have also emerged, with a focus on treating ailments that benefit from the Korean traditional approach to medicine.

Clinics attached to colleges of Korean traditional medicine around the country have been opening up new avenues for treatment with specialized offices for each type of condition. There are centers for arthritis, headaches, allergies, respiratory ailments, strokes, and cancer, as well as clinics for anger and stress management, pediatric care, the four constitutions, and even music therapy. Franchises in the field have also appeared in areas where such treatment is widely recognized to be effective, including obesity, human growth, spinal conditions, sinusitis, atopic dermatitis, and rage. Clinics for detoxification, natural therapy, hair loss treatment, beauty, hearing, and diabetes are also drawing newfound attention. Providers have developed higher quality products, including herbal and facial acupuncture and fermented medicines, as a way of providing more competitive services. At the same time, academic societies have helped turn the clinical experiences of practitioners at university centers and smaller clinics into interesting research findings.

The Korean Traditional Knowledge Portal (www.koreantk.com), which was launched in December 2007, represents a milestone in the promotion of Korean traditional medicine. Administered by the Korean Intellectual Property Office, the website offers a comprehensive database on Korean traditional medicine, including a wide range of categorized information on medicinal ingredients and symptoms, along with access to academic papers. Recent studies and clinical findings of hospitals and universities are continuously posted on the site.

Today, the close collaboration between practitioners of Korean traditional medicine and Western medicine is a truly remarkable development. For example, the East-West Medical Center at Kyung

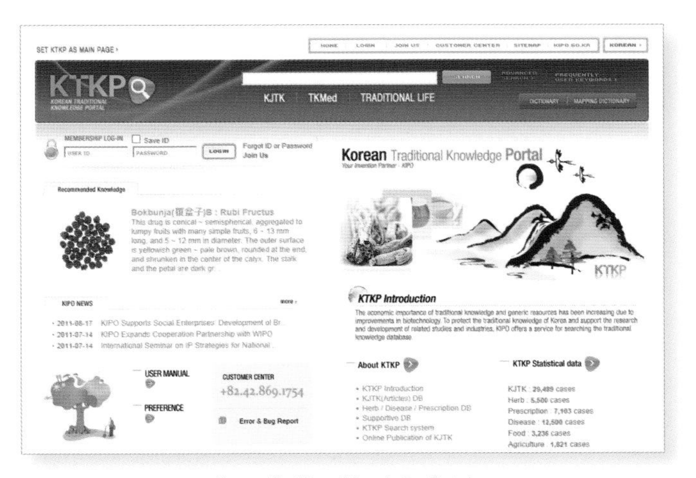

Korean Traditional Knowledge Portal

Hee University Medical Center in Seoul is equipped with state-of-the-art equipment such as CT and MRI units used for a more comprehensive diagnosis, prior to applying traditional treatments such as acupuncture, moxibustion, herbal medicine, and lifestyle management. At such clinics utilizing collaboration between Korean and Western medicine, a patient is evaluated and treated by a joint team of Western and traditional medicine practitioners who can complement each other's specialties. Surgery is done when needed and traditional treatments are prescribed for overall health enhancement.

One example of this cooperation is the treatment of allergic rhinitis. Patients often have problems with their nasal structure. After surgery on the nose is performed at the East-West Medical Center's rhinitis clinic, doctors determine which substance is causing the allergic reaction. The patient receives both acupuncture and treatment with those allergens, which are gradually introduced into the body to build immunity. In this case, the surgery and immune treatment are performed by a Western medicine specialist, while the acupuncture is done by a doctor of Korean traditional medicine. Center director Cho Joong-saeng explains that this combined approach offers a "distinctive system of treatment that can be developed greatly by Koreans, with their long history of traditional medicine."

Recently, the stroke and brain disease center at Kyung Hee University Hospital at Gangdong published significant findings in an international journal on a treatment combining neurosurgery with internal treatment using Korean traditional medicine. When artery walls weaken or arteries are expanded or altered by increased pressure, patients undergoing treatment sometimes exhibit symptoms of stiffness in their extremities and twitching from the pulling of blood vessels. These symptoms are temporary, but with no suitable treatment options available, patients are known to endure great discomfort. The center found visible improvements when patients were given acupuncture on their arms and legs. This study was an opportunity to use Korean traditional medicine to treat symptoms that Western medicine is ineffective against, as well as for Western and Korean physicians alike to observe the effects of medical treatment from a Western perspective.

Universities and think tanks are also conducting diverse research on medicinal herbs and beneficial food ingredients. Folk remedies, which have long been dismissed as simply superstitious or mystic beliefs, are now being reassessed from a scientific approach. This development has resulted in new treatment methods. Through the further integration of Western and traditional medicine practices, a bright outlook lies ahead for the future of Korean traditional medicine.

Modern Diagnostic Equipment

In addition to the four methods outlined in Chapter 3—visual examination, listening/smelling, inquiry, and palpation—doctors of Korean traditional medicine have also been making more use of modern equipment to develop more quantitative and objective forms of treatment.

One example is infrared equipment to examine body heat. Minute amounts of infrared radiation are detected and

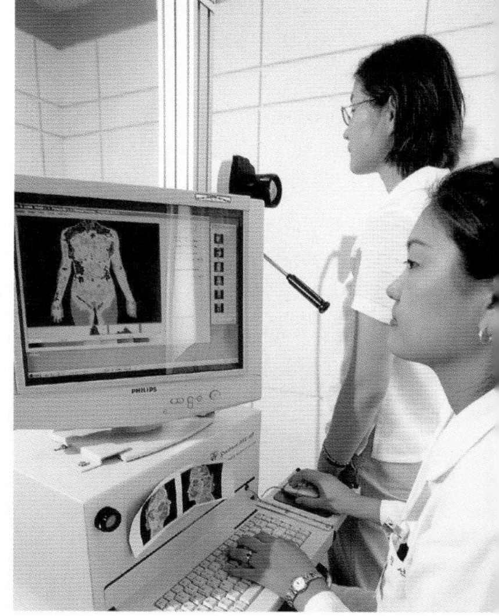

Korean traditional medicine clinics today have advanced equipment for more accurate diagnosis and treatment.

developed into color images that show tiny changes in heat in afflicted areas, helping to locate any abnormalities and diagnose ailments. This objective and non-invasive method can be applied in nervous and musculoskeletal system disorders.

Computerized equipment can also help physicians distinguish the four constitutions and the associated causes of disease. For instance, the *soeum* type is prone to problems with energy circulation and back pain from diminished uterine function, while the *soyang* type is often characterized by lower back problems associated with weak kidney function. The equipment helps the physician to isolate these causes.

Other equipment is used for the diagnostic method known as Ryodoraku. This technique uses electro-conductive lines linked to points in the body where electricity flows are particularly strong. By running a weak current through the body, flows that vary in indirect proportion to resistance in the skin can be observed. These values are shown on a monitor, displaying the skin's resistance to electric currents coming in from outside. Ryodoraku lines are closely linked to the autonomous nervous system and show internal changes to internal organs from the sensory, motor, and autonomous nerves on the body's surface. By using electrical phenomena to observe changes in nervous functions, doctors can observe the functions of certain organs.

The leading methods of stroke diagnosis include the testing of meridian function and examinations of pulse waves and strength. In meridian testing, the body's biorhythms are analyzed to determine the balance of the autonomous nervous system and degree of physical activity. Through this approach, doctors can estimate the degree of aging, stress, and brain activity. One test, the *suyangming* meridian function examination, involves attaching a sensor to the tip of the second finger on the right hand to observe the wavelengths. The doctor can examine the adjustment capabilities

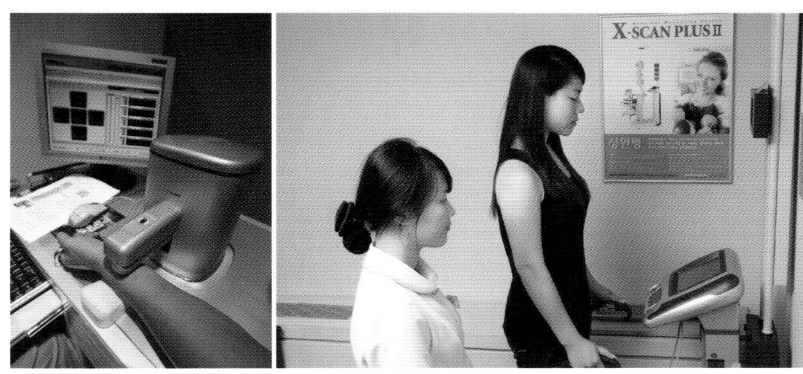

Patient diagnosis with a pulse graph (left) and body composition analyzer (right)

and balance of the autonomous nervous system, while offering calculations of blood vessel elasticity and aging to help stroke prevention.

Pulse wave analysis studies blood to estimate the strength of heart ejection and the elasticity of peripheral blood vessels. By calculating the age of the vessels, doctors can estimate the degree of artery hardening and deterioration, helping to prevent ailments such as hypertension and renal insufficiency.

Pulse graphs are state-of-the-art devices used in Korean traditional medicine to show pulse strength in graph form. They allow the observation of the harmony of energy and blood in the body and the presence of functional problems in the five viscera and six bowels.

Other equipment includes the iris monitor, which is used to observe changes in the body manifested in the eyes. This helps doctors see changes in organs and diagnose their relative health. Another device, used primarily to treat obesity, examines body composition by estimating body fat and muscle.

Globalizing Korean Traditional Medicine

Oriental medicine has attracted growing interest in the West. In the U.S., hundreds of millions of dollars have been allocated for research through the National Center for Complementary and Alternative Medicine to encourage studies in Oriental medicine. Surveys show that around 70 percent of Americans have had experience with Eastern treatment such as acupuncture. Rising interest in natural therapeutics in Europe has led to more spending on non-pharmacological therapies such as acupuncture and yoga. In Germany, the government is leading an initiative to collect natural substances to develop natural drugs; more than 50,000 medical doctors practice both Western and Oriental medicine in that country, acupuncture has grown popular, and a range of Oriental medicine therapies are being practiced. In the U.K., the national acupuncture association has thousands of members. This growing interest has helped Korean traditional medicine reach people all over the world, with colleges springing up at universities in the U.S. and Europe.

Researchers have also tried combining the findings of Western and Korean traditional medicine. In June 2012, the Korea Institute of Oriental Medicine signed a memorandum of understanding to build a technology exchange framework with the Martinos Center for Biomedical Imaging at Harvard University/Massachusetts General Hospital in Boston. The two institutions agreed to cooperate in researcher exchanges, joint research, technology information sharing, symposiums, and seminars. The agreement is expected to contribute to the convergence of Eastern and Western medicine by shedding light on the biological phenomena associated with Korean traditional medications and methods, including acupuncture, moxibustion, and herbal remedies.

What explains the growing global interest in Korean traditional

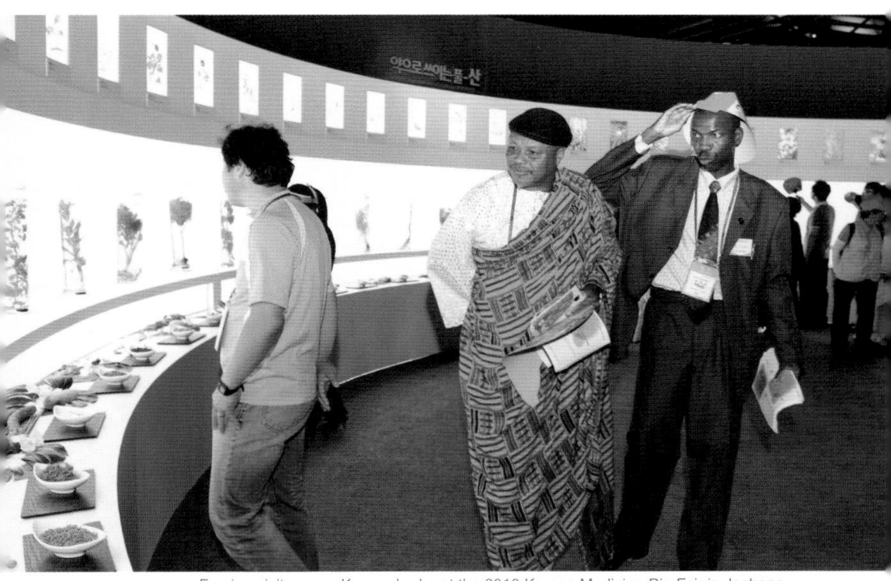

Foreign visitors see Korean herbs at the 2010 Korean Medicine-Bio Fair in Jecheon.

medicine? The first factor is increasing awareness of the limits of the Western approach. Western medicine has contributed much to human health, but is far from the perfect remedy for every disease. Other paradigms are needed to make up for where it falls short. While Western medicine focuses on the visible, Korean traditional medicine looks at functional things that cannot always be seen.

The second factor is knowledge of the side effects of surgical intervention. When a patient undergoes an operation, he or she is unlikely to be the same as before even after recovery is complete. Many patients also have negative reactions to anesthesia and other complications from Western treatment.

The third factor is the growing risks associated with pharmaceuticals, including rejection, resistance, and buildup. A surprising number of patients experience negative side effects to certain types of medicine. Many also develop resistance over long periods of time, which reduces the effectiveness of the treatment. The damages from buildup can be greater still. For example, a person who takes adrenocorticotrophic hormones for chronic neuropathy may recover, but prolonged use can lead to osteoporosis.

International Experiences

What do Wilhelm Donko and Leandro Arellano have in common? Both are former ambassadors to Korea—Donko from Austria, Arellano from Mexico—and also devotees of Korean traditional medicine. They discovered the effects of Korean traditional medicine many years ago when Donko was plagued by sudden back pain and Arellano by neck disc pain, and have come back to clinics for more.

The two diplomats are among a growing number of patients from abroad who frequent clinics of Korean traditional medicine. According to figures from the Korean Ministry of Health and Welfare, the number of foreign patients at such clinics has risen 110.8 percent since 2009. Most hail from Russia and Japan, though many others are from the U.S., Germany, Mongolia, and China. Such patients cite the availability of alternatives to surgery, including acupuncture, herbal remedies, and other physical treatments, as reasons for choosing Korean traditional medicine.

What kind of treatment do they receive? According to Raimund Royer, an Austrian-born doctor of Korean traditional medicine who heads the international clinic at the Jaseng Hospital of Oriental Medicine in Seoul, most seek non-surgical disc treatment. "They've been very satisfied," he says. "The effects of treatment have been enhanced with acupuncture, herbal remedies, and independently developed chuna therapy methods, and it costs

The fourth factor is growing demand for natural treatments for environmental hormones. Modernization has introduced threats to health in food culture in the form of harmful compounds in ingredients and utensils. People want to protect themselves from pesticides and other harmful chemicals. Many have turned to more natural food products and herbal remedies. Korean traditional medicine offers diagnoses and treatments for ailments that have baffled Western medicine—and more people around the world are taking notice.

less than surgery."

Jaseng specializes in spinal problems and has drawn attention by developing effective non-surgical treatment for disc ailments. This has resulted in a rise of 84.6 percent in treatment effects for discs in the lower back, as well as patented new materials for regenerating spinal bones.

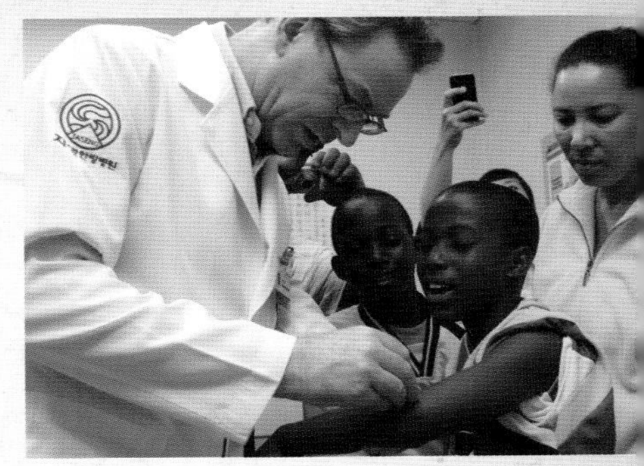

Raimund Royer performs acupuncture on a member of the South African youth soccer team.

The number of international patients going to this clinic is growing. To date, more than 3,000 have visited for treatment. Jaseng now has clinics in eight U.S. locations, including Los Angeles and Fullerton, California, and in New Jersey. Many top hospitals are also showing interest in Jaseng's motion-style acupuncture and Oriental medicine treatments, including the Olympia Medical Center and Cedars-Sinai Medical Center in Los Angeles, St. Jude Medical in Irvine, and Rush University Medical Center in Chicago. These centers are now developing combined East-West approaches in treatment.

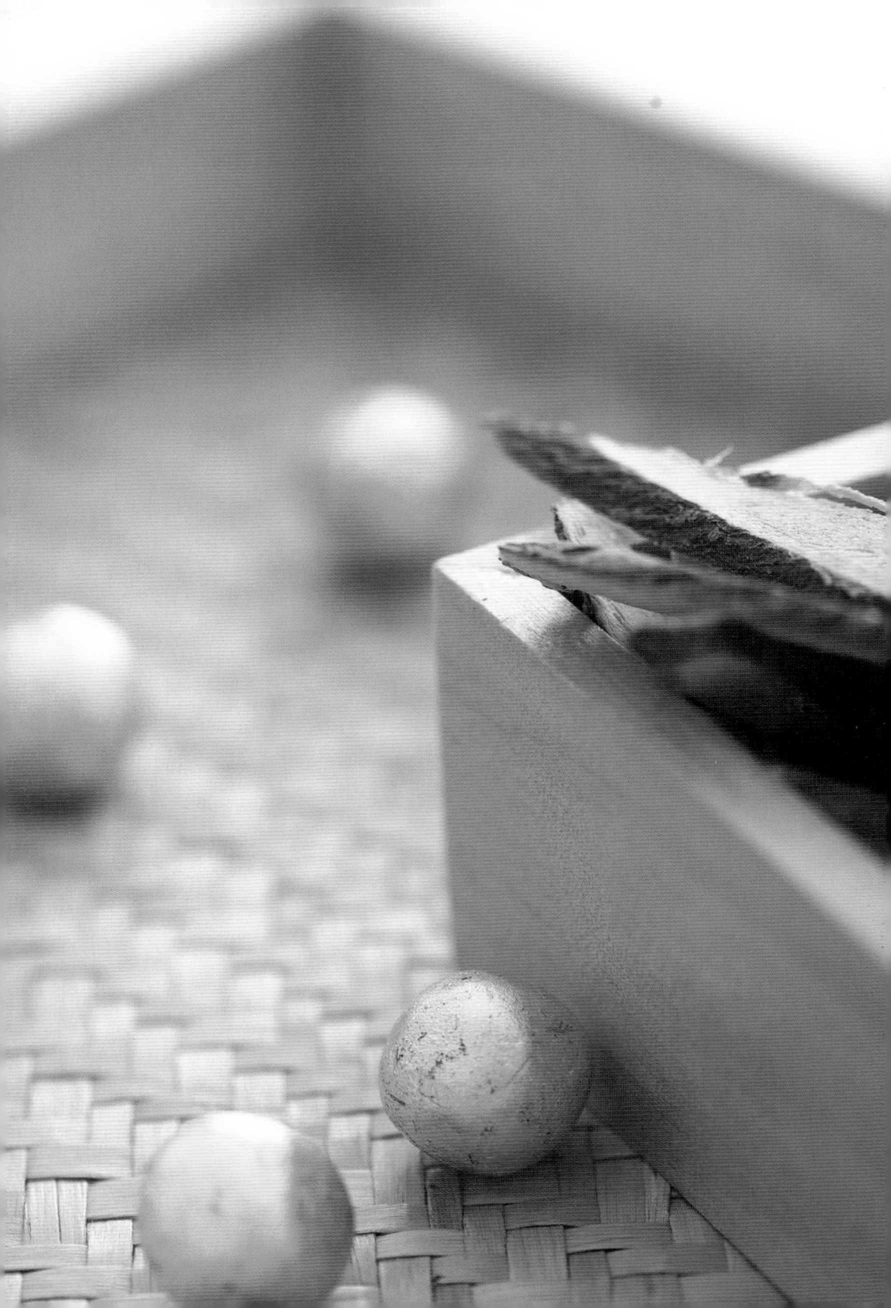

APPENDIX

INFORMATION

Museums

SANCHEONG MUSEUM OF HERBAL MEDICINE

- **Hour** 9am to 6pm. Closed Mondays, New Year's Day, Seollal and Chuseok.
- **Admission** Adults (19-64): 2,000 won / Students (13-18): 1,500 won / Youths (7-12): 1,000 won
- **Address** Donguibogam-ro 555, Geumseo-myeon, Sancheong-gun, Gyeongsangnam-do
- **Tel** +82-55-970-6431~2
- Reservations for foreigners are available.
- **Website** museum.sancheong.ne.kr

DAEGU YANGNYEONGSI ORIENTAL MEDICINE CULTURAL CENTER

- **Hour** 10am to 6pm. Closed Mondays, New Year's Day, Seollal and Chuseok.
- **Admission** Free (Some hands-on programs require admission fees.)
- **Address** 49, Dalgubeol-daero 415-gil, Jung-gu, Daegu, Gyeongsangbuk-do
- **Tel** +82-53-253-3359
- Reservations are required for the group of 10 or more people.
- Audio guides are provided in 4 languages: Korean, English, Japanese and Chinese.
- **Website** dgom.daegu.go.kr/eng

SEOUL YANGNYEONGSI HERB MEDICINE MUSEUM

- **Hour** 10am to 6pm (Mar to Oct), 10am to 5pm (Nov to Feb). Closed Mondays, New Year's Day, Seollal and Chuseok.
- **Admission** Free (Some hands-on programs require admission fees.)
- **Address** 128, Wangsan-ro, Dongdaemun-gu, Seoul
- **Tel** +82-2-3293-4900~3
- Reservations are required for the group of 20 or more people.
- Prior reservation is required for the guide.
- **Website** museum.ddm.go.kr

HEOJUN MUSEUM

- **Hour** 10am to 6pm (Mar to Oct), 10am to 5pm (Nov to Feb, weekends and holidays). Closed Mondays, New Year's Day, Seollal and Chuseok.
- **Admission** Adults (19-64): 800 won / Youths (7-18): 500 won
- **Address** 87, Heojun-ro, Gangseo-gu, Seoul
- **Tel** +82-2-3661-8686
- Reservations are required for the group of 20 or more people.
- **Website** www.heojun.seoul.kr

USEFUL WEBSITES

- Korean Traditional Knowledge Portal www.koreantk.com/en
- The Association of Korean Medicine www.akom.org/eng
- Korea Institute of Oriental Medicine www.kiom.re.kr/eng
- All That Korean Medicine tkmedicine.blogspot.kr

The content of this book has been compiled, edited, and supplemented by Hur Inn-hee based on the following articles published in:

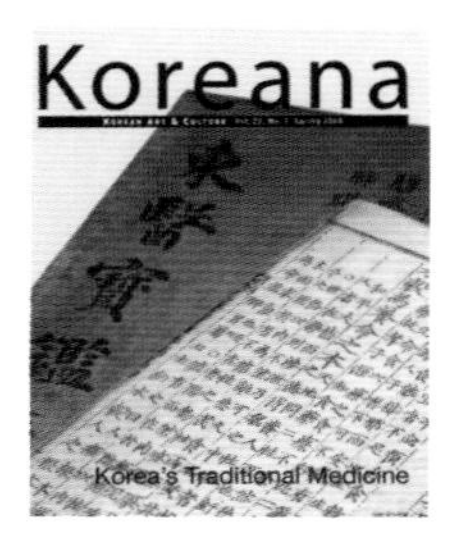

***KOREANA*, Vol.22, No.1, Spring 2000**
"Introduction to Korea Traditional Medicine"
by Shin Joon-shik

"Three Popular Applications of Korea Traditional Medicine"
by Ko Changnam

"Outlook for Korea Traditional Medicine"
by Chae Yoon-jung

Chapter 2,3 and 5 were newly written by Hur Inn-hee.

PHOTOGRAPHS

Korea Tourism Organization 18, 24, 41, 45, 47, 49, 63, 65, 66, 67, 82, 87,
Chunwondang Museum of Korean Medicine 34
Seo Heun-kang 14, 55
Ryu Seung-hoo 13, 60
Yonhap Photo 13, 15, 16, 17, 24, 42, 75, 81, 89, 91
Newsbank Image 79, 85
Image Today 5, 7, 8, 11, 27, 33, 50, 51, 54, 57, 58, 59, 62, 64, 69, 71, 73, 76, 92
Topic Image 21

Credits

Publisher	Kim Hyung-geun
Writer	Hur Inn-hee
Translator	Colin A. Mouat
Editor	Kim Eugene
Copy Editor	D. Peter Kim
Designer	Jung Hyun-young